Advance P1
Be Your Own Superhero

"Barbara's compelling journey through chronic disease provides all of us a road map and resources to overcome adversity."

— *Richard Carmona, MD, MPH, FACS; 17th Surgeon General of the United States; Distinguished Professor, University of Arizona*

"Only someone who has lived and breathed a disease can truly know what it feels like from the inside out. Barbara tells her own powerful story and the stories of others facing major life changing challenges with the insight that can only come from personal experience. Not only does she share all that she's learned on her transforming and courageous journey, but she shares her priceless, powerful tools. Honest, authentic, life affirming and thoroughly inspiring, she shares her amazing G.I.F.T."

— *Franne Golde – wife, mother, advocate, Grammy-Award-nominated songwriter, and founder of frannegolde.com*

"From her own personal journey of resilience, Barbara writes with candor, compassion, and hope about responding to adversity with tenacity, purpose, and grace. In a captivating, warm style, she provides specific, actionable steps for building resilience and wellness. This book has universal appeal, as its tools are pertinent not only to individuals living with multiple sclerosis but also to individuals facing other challenges, whether they are chronic illness, loss, or everyday stressors."

"Barbara Appelbaum's writing is smart, detailed and informative. *Be Your Own Superhero* is a true look at multiple sclerosis (and other chronic disease) and a guidebook for others to feel in control of both the disease and the many facets of living a full life."

"We are all superheroes! With great power comes great responsibility. (First stated by Voltaire and recently attributed to Stan Lee in *Spider-Man*). We must each own these responsibilities – eat to live instead of living to eat. Remember to adequately nourish, hydrate and use our bodies in ways in which they are meant to be challenged daily through exercise and rest – intellectually and through meditation. Avoid vices such as smoking, illicit drugs and over-medication, excessively drinking alcohol, and obesity. Enjoy the outdoors, nature and other creatures and spend as much time traveling as a native as you do as a tourist. Learn the benefits and wisdom of other cultures and our ancestors. Learn to listen to your own body. Check in with your health care team regularly and educate yourself about your predisposition to illness, both genetically and environmentally, and become proactive. Remember, when you stop growing and learning, you start dying. Don't forget that every day above ground is a great day, and live each one to its fullest. Don't just exist through life. Make a difference in the world by generously giving of yourself; the rewards are immense. Don't settle with being ordinary; choose to be extraordinary. The choices we each make are powerful and affect the long-term outcome of how we will enjoy our lives as we age. *Make great choices and enjoy living a meaningful life!!! Use your superpowers wisely.* Barbara illustrates the importance of acquisition of tools to facilitate all of the aforementioned, despite life's unexpected adversities."

— *Clara Raquel Epstein, MD, FICS; Neurosurgeon/CEO, The Epstein Neurosurgery Center, LLC, The Epstein Neurosurgery Foundation, Inc. 501(c)(3), "Exceptional Neurosurgical Care"*

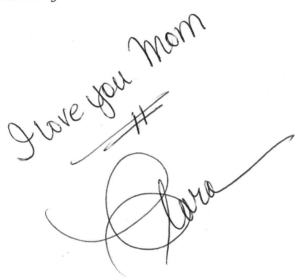

Be Your Own Superhero

A Road Map to Resilience when Faced with Chronic Dis-ease

Barbara B. Appelbaum, PCC, MBA, MAT

Author of *Live in Wellness Now:*
A Proactive Guide to Living Well

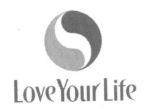

Love Your Life

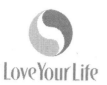
Love Your Life

Author photo by R.C. Clark Dancing Snake Nature Photography

Author Contact: http://appelbaumwellness.com

Love Your Life Publishing

Wilmington, DE

ISBN: 978-1-934509-93-7

Library of Congress Control Number: 2018935320

Printed in the United States of America

First Printing: 2018

Editing by Gwen Hoffnagle

Cover Design by Sarah Barrie of Cyanotype.ca

To protect the privacy of individuals, groups and/or places discussed, names and identifying details have been changed or were purposely unspecified.

This book is not intended to be a substitute for the medical advice of a licensed physician. The reader should consult with their doctor regarding any matters relating to their health.

She needed a hero; so she became one.

— Anonymous

And God said to me:

"Believe in yourself; you are the change you wish to see in the world.
You help others navigate their path through pain to wellness.
You make other people's lives easier, you make a difference.
You matter. Just breathe. Trust in your journey. Trust the process.
All is as it is meant to be.
I choose you because you can handle it. Now teach others.
Remember, I AM..."

– Barbara B. Appelbaum

(Personal reflections on what inspired me to write this book.)

TABLE OF CONTENTS

Hardships often prepare ordinary people for an extraordinary destiny.

– C. S. Lewis

The Road Less Traveled: My Message to Multiple Sclerosis after Diagnosis

You entered my life out of the blue in 2006, like a freight train derailing at top speed, and changed everything. You put me on the road less traveled; one that I would have ignored otherwise. As much as I tried to stay the course of my normal existence, you pushed me in the direction of another – the one truly meant for me even though I didn't recognize it at the time.

As I navigated this new life path, you tried with all your might to knock me down, but I refused to fall. Through your challenging lessons you have shown me that I am not weak but strong; not hopeless but determined; and not diseased but healthy for me. You have become an integral part of me and although I occasionally stumble, I always pick myself up, dust myself off and start anew. You may always be the proverbial "elephant in the room" but I have learned to look past your oversized body and see everything else for the blessings they are.

When you first came into my life many people asked me, "Why you?" and my reply was simple: "Because I can handle it." I find your entering my life to be the greatest gift I ever received. You awakened within me a strength I didn't realize I had and taught me to live the life I want, not the one others think I should. You taught me a greater empathy for others who live their lives in constant suffering and gave me the tools to pass on my knowledge to help them be their own best advocates in order to live well. You also taught me what I have known all along even though I didn't consciously realize it: when chaos arrives at my front door I do not panic. I respond with resilience.

Learning to overcome adversity is truly one of life's gifts. When faced with a challenge there is always an opportunity that lies within that can be discovered by Getting clear, Increasing understanding, Focusing and Taking action (G.I.F.T.). You offered me an opportunity, and through it I discovered my purpose of being and am able to live my best, healthiest life. Thanks to you I have come into my own. And although it is a long road to accepting and coming to terms with your existence, I know I have the courage and faith necessary to thrive.

Through my story I will teach others how to navigate their life's journey to their best ability by sharing how I traverse each step, each stumble and each giant leap, walking together down the path of life, taking that road less traveled.

PREFACE

———

BE PRESENT

In the middle of difficulty lies opportunity.
– Albert Einstein

Imagine standing at the edge of an ocean, mesmerized by the ebb and flow of the waves. Some gently lap against the rocks; others come in more forcefully. Regardless of strength, the waves come in and then roll back out to sea. Countless living organisms ride this continuous cycle along with your body as if the energy of the earth is in sync with your breath by means of the motion of the water. As you watch the waves and witness the vast strength of the water, you are in awe. Awe is an emotion combining dread, reverence and wonder that is inspired by the sacred or magnificent. As you stand at the water's edge soaking in this magnificence, you innately understand there must be a power greater than you, whether you call it God, Spirit, Energy or something else.

As you become present to the moment, you trust in your higher power and imagine casting the negative thoughts and feelings that weigh you down into the sea. Recognize that you are but one small component in this infinite universe. Open yourself up to receive positive energy, helping you focus on your breath, nourishing your body, mind and spirit.

In order to be, one must do. I believe a person's life is about being the change they want to see in the world. It is about walking your talk every day through helping and truly listening to others with a nonjudgmental approach. It is about being kind and expressing gratitude. This, in turn, reflects in your overall wellness. Life teaches you to be the cause of your existence, not the effect, and that only you can shift your way of thinking to transform your feelings and behavior. This is the purpose of your superhero journey.

Imagine feeling the breeze gently blowing through your hair and the warmth of the sunshine on your face. Notice the bees pollinating the wildflowers around the rocks, continuing the cycle of life. What type of person will you become as you mature? What impact will you have in this world, and will it be lasting? In what way will the world be better off for your having been in it? Your mind might be filled with rhetorical questions about your own humanity to which only God/ Spirit/Energy knows the answers as you endeavor to uncover them. Listen to the universe; listen to and trust your instinct. Become present to the moment.

Now imagine sitting in a stark examination room being told of a dreaded diagnosis. Whether serious or minor, it is quite the surprise, immediately aging you as it sends shockwaves throughout your entire nervous system, thrusting your subconscious into questioning the validity of it all. Yet somewhere deep inside you a quiet voice persists with the poignant message that all will be okay.

This is something I don't have to imagine because over a decade ago my life changed in this way forever, in what seemed like the blink of an eye. After experiencing symptoms similar to those of a stroke, I received a diagnosis of multiple sclerosis (MS). And as unusual as this might sound, it was a gift. I know you may be thinking, "Is she nuts?" But all I can say is at the time I was simply going through the motions of my life, and this diagnosis woke me up to actually living my life and becoming present to the moment, which helped me discover my superpowers of resilience and courage. As your illness or problem becomes familiar – unique to you and to your capabilities of handling it, on some level you begin to focus on a solution (perhaps without consciously knowing it). This challenge becomes your steppingstone to discovering new opportunities as well as your inner strength and confidence.

Life is filled with struggle and ease, deterioration and restoration. As you wrestle to live a life of meaning, you will most likely be thwarted by illness brought on by stress or simply due to aging. You cannot escape this fate, but you can learn to bravely stare it in the face until it cowers. When you do this you end up creating a new identity – a more confident sense of self. To get to that point you will likely experience a rite of passage through the five stages of grief: denial, anger, bargaining, depression and acceptance, after which you will make sense of your own unique existence, valuing the preciousness and fragility of life.

The older we get, the years seemingly fly by faster and faster. This is why it is super important to make the most of every minute and not waste precious moments. MS presents issues that can interfere with my daily life. Although I walk a very challenging journey, I share the promise that there is hope and that you can live joyously with chronic disease or "dis-ease." With that said, I continually ask the lingering question, "How well will I be as I age?" After all, aging is inevitable, but how you age is not. People with illnesses that are not chronic usually either experience remission, are healed, or pass away – a bit more finite than my experience with MS. People like me with chronic disease learn to live with their illnesses by making friends with the proverbial elephant in the room who never leaves. Regardless, everyone has something; life goes on until it doesn't; and you do the best you can along the way.

Have you ever just sat and thought, "Damn, I've been through a lot of sh*t"? As you reflected, you probably recognized the gravity of all you have experienced – the good and the bad. Be grateful for the amazing life you have and all the opportunities that come with it. We live life on autopilot so much that it becomes normal; therefore we don't consciously recognize we're doing it. Yet when you turn off your autopilot, even if only fleetingly, you become present to the moment and discover how you have grown and what you have learned over time. You shift to "possibility thinking": envisioning living well and enjoying a meaningful life.

My life is abundant with blessings. If I were to measure wealth by the number of blessings I have, I am one of the richest people on earth. Yet I've had my fair share of obstacles, which is part of a person's normal human existence. The major traumatic events I have experienced are being a victim of bullying at a young age, the death of my true love, a bad marriage that ended in divorce, and two devastating diagnoses. As I wrote this book I took a moment to reread letters and emails that family and close friends wrote to me when I was first impacted by several of these life-altering ordeals. I was struck by the common theme among them all: everyone considered me to be a resilient, tough, good person who always put others first, stating that I was the epitome of "when bad things happen to good people."

Rabbi Harold Kushner wrote a book called *When Bad Things Happen to Good People*, in which he discussed the difference between God intervening in our lives and the power of free will. He stated that God does not pick and choose what happens to us; it is our own free will that determines our destiny. Never have I blamed God for any of the adversities in my life. You might think that I'm not being honest with myself; after all, doesn't everyone cry out, "Why me?" to God/Spirit/Energy when the proverbial rug is pulled out from under them? As I've matured and developed my emotional strength, I choose to say, "Why not me?" because no one is to blame for what has happened to me, not even myself. And perhaps everything truly does happen for a reason.

I alone am responsible for how I respond to such events. And thanks to my upbringing and lessons learned from a childhood game, my parents taught me to respond with resilience. Although at times I may feel broken, hopeless or scared, I have learned that I am powerful beyond measure when I tap into my superpower of resilience. Resilience empowers me to be in control of my health instead of being a victim of it. It creates abundance and wholeness. There are several ways to build or nurture your resilience: shifting your mindset, exchanging negative self-talk for positive self-talk, coping, socializing, discovering your purpose or passion in life, exercising, eating nutritious food, and having a spirituality practice. Resilience exists within you; you simply must cultivate it so as to strengthen it.

The Miriam-Webster dictionary defines *resilience* as "the ability to become strong, healthy, or successful again after something bad happens." It is the capacity to move forward even in the face of adversity, chronic stress, anger, fear, grief or sadness. Most people possess some degree of resilience and are able to turn hardship into triumph while discovering that happiness comes from within (or, as I like to say, happiness is an inside job). Strengthening your resilience is not always easy; it takes hard work. And along the way it is okay to cry, be angry or be vulnerable. Just remember to laugh and let go once in a while. Trust yourself to adapt to circumstances, which affords you the space to thrive. Adversity happens to you; it does not define who you are.

I recently read in a Jewish National Fund newsletter that the Hebrew verb for overcoming an adversity, *lehitgaber*, is commonly used when describing success against a challenge. I was happily surprised to learn that the Hebrew root of that verb – consisting of the Hebrew letters *gimel*, *bet* and *resh* – is also the foundation for the Hebrew word *gibor*, meaning hero. Add this to the idea that superhero stories inspire us by providing models of coping with misfortune, discovering our life's purpose, and uncovering our strengths and using them for good. Therefore it is not far-reaching to conclude that when you overcome adversity using your superpower of resilience, you become your own superhero, able to live well with chronic disease or chronic dis-ease.

Let's face it; we are all aging, which is a good thing! And if you are part of the Baby Boomer generation like me, you might feel great in midlife but might not be as physically well as you actually feel. According to an article in *AARP The Magazine* there was a landmark study called "Midlife in the United States" that revealed "people in their 50s say they feel ten years younger than their physical age yet, according to the Centers for Disease Control and Prevention (CDC), have a heart that functions as if it were in its 60s."[1] Feeling 10 years younger but having the heart of someone 10 years older is simply not good. Combine this data with the fact that many put off seeing a doctor for physicals and prescribed wellness checks including colonoscopy and other cancer screenings, as well as become more sedentary, opening the door for unwanted weight gain, forgetfulness and the need for medication to control things like high blood pressure and cholesterol. And according to my gynecologist, age is the number one risk factor for developing cancer. If you are in Generation X or the Millennial generation, statistics show that you are more technology-focused and work-oriented, so you lead a more sedentary lifestyle than others, with greater stress and feelings of responsibility, which contribute to having more health issues than others. So why are so many of us managing our "sick care" instead of being proactive about our health care?

According to the National Council on Health, more than 133 million Americans (over 40 percent of the population) have at least one chronic condition.[2] This book is written in response to this alarming statistic and for the 76 million Baby Boomers,

65 million Gen Xers, and 85 million Millennials who may already have a chronic illness or age-related health issue and are eager for practical and sage advice on how you, although not responsible for getting sick, can learn to be your healthiest self. In general, *Be Your Own Superhero* is for anyone who wants to be proactive about disease prevention, health and well-being, and develop simple but extraordinary health practices for longevity, even with a chronic disease.

As we journey together in *Be Your Own Superhero*, I ask that you reflect on your life experiences, especially in regard to your personal health and wellness. No matter your age or health, have faith that even if you are feeling distress or are limited, together we will discover your superpowers of courage and resilience so that you, too, can tap into your unlimited potential, find wholeness and joyously be your own superhero.

INTRODUCTION

THE SUPERHERO JOURNEY

My dear, you always had the power within you.
– Glenda the Good Witch, in The Wizard of Oz

As a kid, did you ever wish you could meet a superhero – or better yet, become one? If you've just received a diagnosis of a chronic and/or age-related illness, I bet you wish you had superpowers to heal yourself. Hold tight, because your wish is about to come true!

To establish a starting point let's begin with answering the key question "What is health?" According to the World Health Organization, "Health is a state of complete physical, mental and social well-being and not merely the absence of disease or infirmity."[3] The National Wellness Institute defines wellness as "an active process through which people become aware of, and make choices towards, a more successful existence."[4] Health and wellness are the foundations of a successful life: the coming together of mind, body and spirit in a harmony that is unique to you. Take note: nowhere in the definitions of health and wellness is the word *disease* used. You can achieve health and wellness even in the presence of illness, because they involve the integrated balance of your physical, emotional and spiritual energy within your body.

The origin of the word *disease* is rooted in Latin and means lack of ease or discomfort. Medically speaking, the term *disease* represents a group of symptoms assigned a specific name. For example, sneezing, coughing, watery eyes and a scratchy throat grouped together are termed a cold. Disease can also be interpreted as dis-ease. The term *dis-ease* means a lack of ease or congruence in your body – a lack of wellness. (From here forward I write "chronic disease" for simplicity, but please keep in mind that what I write refers equally to chronic dis-ease.)

According to the U.S. National Center for Health Statistics, "Chronic disease is one lasting 3 months or more," and that "generally cannot be prevented by vaccines or cured by medication, nor does it just disappear."[5] According to the Centers for Disease Control and Prevention, "Seven of the top 10 causes of death in 2014 were chronic diseases," and "Eighty-six percent of the nation's $2.7 trillion annual heath care expenditures are for people with chronic and mental health conditions."[6] And "chronic diseases affect approximately 133 million Americans, representing more than 40% of the total population of this country. By 2020, that number is projected to grow to an estimated 157 million," according to the National Health Council.[7] A few examples of chronic disease are heart disease, obesity, Alzheimer's and other dementias, arthritis, asthma and autoimmune diseases like MS and lupus, many of which are invisible diseases (in which a person can look healthy regardless of their actual health).

A primary contributor to disease is chronic stress. Stress, good and bad, is everywhere. Good stress is marked by feelings of exhilaration or excitement. Bad stress can shroud you in turmoil. Many people are overloaded with stress every day, operating in crisis mode as a way of life. Research reveals that chronic stress takes a toll on the immune system, weakening it and making the body more susceptible to illness and diminished brain health. How one experiences and copes with stress varies widely from person to person.

Stress is a measure of your body's resistance to real or perceived threats or circumstances beyond your control – your *fight or flight* response. Simply put, it is your body's survival mechanism. Whether it takes the form of excitement, anxiety or fear, it can manifest physically as a rapid pulse, a quick temper, an inability to focus or extreme fatigue, to name just a few symptoms. *Stress* is a word people use frequently in everyday dialogue; "I'm feeling stressed out" is something you might find yourself saying regularly, and when you do I bet you tend to trivialize it, brushing it off like it's a normal part of everyday life. Life, after all, is stressful. However, stress is something to be taken seriously because prolonged symptoms can lead to serious illness and dis-ease.

The brain's fight or flight response mechanism is the physiological response to any perceived threat to survival. According to a Harvard Health Publishing article, "Understanding the Stress Response," "When someone experiences a stressful event, the amygdala, an area of the brain that contributes to emotional processing, sends a distress signal to the hypothalamus. This area of the brain functions like a command center, communicating with the rest of the body through the nervous system so that the person has the energy to fight or flee."[8] In an emergency or during an urgent event such as the sudden onset of illness, the body sends a message of perceived danger to the amygdala and then a distress signal is sent to the hypothalamus. This area of the brain communicates with the rest of the body via the nervous system, which controls heart rate, breathing, blood pressure and so forth. When this mechanism is repeatedly triggered by the multitude of modern-day stressors, the body gets overwhelmed, the immune system is compromised and stress-related illness sets in. Combined with less-than-healthy lifestyle choices, these symptoms can create a ripe environment for chronic illness to take hold. The question *Be Your Own Superhero* will help you answer is how you (or your brain) can best respond to such symptoms to avoid the onset of a chronic illness or live a healthier life with a chronic disease.

> *Whatever you fight, you strengthen. What you resist,*
> *persists. Fear is our friend. Fear is a natural reaction to*
> *moving closer to the truth. Nothing ever goes away until it*
> *has taught us what we need to know.*
> – Pema Chodron

In the US about one quarter of the total population is the Baby Boomer generation – approximately 76 million people make up this aging population that is, understandably, fearful of physical and cognitive decline. Our number one fear is developing Alzheimer's disease, a rapidly accelerating condition and currently the sixth leading cause of death. We are living longer and therefore need strong, agile minds to keep up with and maintain our bodies. The good news is that it is possible to slow down degeneration or even enhance cognitive function through simple lifestyle modifications.

Research reveals via the concept of neuroplasticity that the brain has the capacity to grow stronger as we mature. Once thought to be static or finite, it turns out that our brains, which have the consistency of soft butter, are malleable and can grow new synaptic pathways and neurons throughout our lives. Proper nutrition, exercise, socializing and spiritual practices contribute to the creation of *brain reserve*: the brain's resistance to damage, also known as the brain's resilience. According to positive psychology and neuroscience, the brain's resilience is directly related to developing resilience in ourselves, possibility thinking and positive behavior. Resilience and behavior are directly linked to thoughts and how they affect feelings, and, in turn, how they affect actions. As Buddha states, "What you think, you become. What you feel, you attract. What you imagine, you create."

We are intrigued by superheroes because they are ordinary people doing extraordinary feats. In superheroes we see the promise of our own potential, and we dare to imagine having our own super-capabilities. Superheroes invariably undergo some kind of an ordeal that reveals their strengths and how best to use them. Author and mythologist Joseph Campbell calls this "The Hero's Journey." It's what happens when someone is called from the ordinary world – usually through a discovery, an unexpected event or a trauma – and journeys on a quest. The hero/heroine is thrust into a new, unfamiliar world in which there is treasure and danger, obstacles and allies, trials and gifts, struggle and ease. The journey is always life-changing, and not just for the journeyer: the hero eventually returns home with an elixir that helps others to be extraordinary in their own ordinary life journeys.

My most poignant and significant quest began with an unexpected and devastating health diagnosis at the young age of 44. I received a diagnosis of multiple sclerosis, a lifelong and progressive autoimmune disease that affects more than 2.5 million people worldwide. I was reluctantly thrust into an unknown world, facing many tests and challenges, until gradually this new world became familiar and manageable. I learned to be my own superhero; to find and cultivate the extraordinary qualities within that make me uniquely able to handle what life has given me. And I believe that just as I can be my own superhero, so can you!

So don your virtual cape and strike your favorite power pose, because *Be Your Own Superhero* is the gift I return with – the elixir to help you uncover your own superhero qualities for the challenges you face in life. Whether you are of the Baby Boomer, X, or Millennial generation, it is intended especially for the millions of people living with chronic disease and for the many more millions facing age-related illnesses and dis-ease. It is worth noting, however, that the tools in this book are skills for living well, and that being the best versions of ourselves physically, mentally, emotionally and spiritually is always life-enhancing.

As a result of MS I was inspired to become a health and wellness coach and consultant. Through my work with others over the past decade I have discovered that everyone has their own superhero qualities within, ready to come forward when invited. By combining neuroscience research and spiritual principles, *Be Your Own Superhero* outlines a proactive, four-step process I call G.I.F.T. that shows you how to develop your own best health practices and superhero qualities. I'll explain more about G.I.F.T. in just a bit; for now the most important thing to know is that the rewards from using this process are super-sized and include a sense of empowerment, learning to look beyond limitations, greater self-esteem, clarity concerning personal goals, and the ability to live your healthiest life even with chronic disease!

We live in an imperfect world seen through the filter of what we think should be perfection. And the G.I.F.T. process does not imply that life is about silver linings and seeing the world through rose-colored glasses. Treating disease is not necessarily about healing and recovery; it's about having the tenacity, knowledge and courage to be as healthy as possible. It's about honoring your own perfectly imperfect self.

***

My parents raised me with a strong sense of doing the right thing, being grateful and being a good person. They taught me the Jewish concept of *tikkun olam* – a responsibility to heal and repair the world. I was the youngest of three children and the only girl, and there was always an abundance of love in our home. Lessons handed down to me were rooted in a strong value system: earning what I wanted and understanding I could have anything, just not everything. It was expected that I would grow up to be confident, poised and well-educated so as to marry a man of integrity and wealth with whom to settle down and raise a family. That was easier said than done.

I was bullied incessantly throughout my school years. Bullies found me an easy target because I was shy. My parents never taught me to be tough, only to be sweet and polite – a "good little girl." They also taught me to think, and through games, meaningful conversation and modeling their teachings through their behavior, my critical-thinking skills matured. Over time my street-smart, practical skills of resilience were deeply nurtured and embedded.

Immersing myself in academia afforded me the respite I needed to figure out what I wanted to be when I grew up. Although I found the coursework challenging, I managed to achieve a bachelor's degree and two master's degrees. During my college years I met my soulmate, who was abruptly taken away from me by leukemia when I was just 23 years old. Several years later I married and then divorced. The idyllic dream of a dependable husband, a house in suburbia with a white picket fence, 2.5 kids and a dog eluded me. A lingering shadow of sadness that I had not achieved the stereotypical goals society imposed on me cast a pall over my life.

Throughout much of my life I have felt like a misfit, always being the round peg that so desperately wanted to fit into the square hole. It seemed I could never accomplish the things that were expected of me. Turning 40, I experienced a midlife crisis because I had not achieved my expectations of success. I suffered a major meltdown that catalyzed a desperate quest of researching what I might do to change the miserable feelings that seemed to consume me. Fortunately I worked in the business side of health care, so I had numerous resources readily available to me. I embarked on the inner work of shifting my perspective, focusing deliberately on what I had accomplished instead of what I had not. Slowly I began to feel in control of my life. Receiving the diagnosis of MS in 2006 at the age of 44 shook me again, and subsequently led to not only adjusting to new limitations of my body, but to losing my job, several friends and my childhood dreams of a future I now thought had been taken away from me.

The unpredictability that accompanies living with any chronic disease and its symptoms presented tangible challenges that made me doubt and question myself. *Had I caused my illness?* My neurologist had drawn a direct connection between my health history and my having MS. *Could I have taken better care of myself? Will this dreadful disease cause my life to be cut short?*

However, like a phoenix rising from the ashes, my resilience and faith in myself rose up through the turmoil and I grew strong, emotionally and physically, rebuilding the foundation of well-being I had previously established by shifting my perspective on life and using my childhood training in critical thinking. In the coming pages I will share my journey – from onset to diagnosis to learning to live well with a chronic disease – so that, like me, you can learn to be your own superhero.

I understand completely that no one is responsible or to blame for having an illness – but each of us is responsible for how we live with it. If you are dealing with illness or dis-ease (stress), I want you to know that your response, whatever that is, is perfectly normal and understandable. You are not alone in your thoughts and feelings, and you do have inner heroic resources you may not have even dared to imagine. Together we will discover and cultivate the extraordinary qualities within you that make you uniquely able to cope with whatever life hands you.

There are four phases of growing from adversity to opportunity: trauma, grief, acceptance and thriving. In my signature strategic-thinking process that I will teach you, the four corresponding steps are: 1) Get clear; 2) Increase understanding; 3) Focus; and 4) Take action (G.I.F.T.). When a crisis occurs you can get stuck in the murkiness of questioning why. As a human being it is normal to be consumed with negative thoughts during a time of trauma. Together we will explore how to reframe your thinking to be more positive and adaptable to problematic circumstances. Like your malleable brain, you will learn how to adapt to change without breaking. And you will learn to listen to and trust your inner voice, recognizing that it always knows what is best for you.

Using the principles of neuroscience and spirituality to guide you through proven practices for taking control of your health and life, I will help you discover your superpowers. I will partner with you as we harness my four-step strategic-thinking process to reach deep inside to discover your resilience, exploring the thoughts behind your behaviors to maximize your potential while addressing limitations and considering how you can live well with chronic disease. I will offer suggestions and tips for making small, sustainable choices that lead to remarkable, lasting change. This book is not filled with quick fixes or my telling you what to think or how to behave. *Be Your*

Own Superhero is about embracing your perfectly imperfect self and appreciating your exceptional abilities. A lot of information will be disseminated. To avoid overwhelm, pick out one or two nuggets that speak directly to you and implement them. Over time continue to add in what works for you and weed out what does not.

My childhood lessons, along with the hurdles I have traversed over the years, taught me how to cope and be resilient. As my father's favorite philosophical quote by Robert Elias states, "If you can't fight and you can't flee; flow." As we journey together in *Be Your Own Superhero* you will discover your "flow," decrease stress, increase your ability to cope, shift your thinking from fear to resilience to healing, and learn how to live well with chronic disease. You will be able to joyously respond to the question "How alive am I willing to be?"

Wellness Self-Assessment

Let's face it; everyone has something. And that something usually becomes more abundant with age. Whether it's chronic disease or dis-ease, you most likely are experiencing some sort of disconnect in your life that causes you stress and/or diminished vitality. Even with this happening, you can be your own superhero! You possess many superpowers that you might not notice because you haven't taken the time to reflect on yourself. So before we begin your superhero journey, let's take a moment to tap into how you feel right now at this very minute, putting you and your awareness of self at the top of your priority list.

Do you often ask, "Is this all there is?" allowing stress, worry or fear to make you sick? Do you wish you could wake up each day feeling energized, motivated and focused on living out your dreams? Do you perhaps look in the mirror every morning and not recognize who is looking back at you?

To discover what areas of your life might be holding you back from living purposefully and well, please complete the following wellness self-assessment by marking the statements that are true for you right now. I urge you not to overthink this and to try to accurately portray what is typical for you.

Goals

- ☐ Compared to what I dreamed of when young, I feel I am on track with my goals.
- ☐ My life is meaningful and important to me.
- ☐ I am an active participant in my life, doing what I've always envisioned and not waiting for something to happen.
- ☐ As I grow older, I have plenty of activities and interests to keep me engaged, happy and learning.
- ☐ If today were my last, I'd have no regrets and feel as if I lived a full, purposeful life on my terms.

Relationships

- ☐ I am happy with my relationship status (married, dating, single, etc.).
- ☐ I have many close friends.
- ☐ My family and friends appreciate me.
- ☐ I enjoy hanging out with my family and friends.
- ☐ I surround myself with positive, energetic people who do not drain me.

Career/Work

- ☐ My career/work is fulfilling and I look forward to going to work every day.
- ☐ My skills are put to good use at work.
- ☐ My work responsibilities are clear.
- ☐ My colleagues respect me and my expertise.
- ☐ My values are aligned with those at my place of employment.

☐ I feel valued and optimistic when at work.

☐ When conflict arises at work, I am confident it is handled with fairness.

Self-Care/Wellness

☐ I exercise at least three or four times a week.

☐ I live a balanced life, getting enough sleep and working eight hours a day or less.

☐ I eat healthfully, avoiding too much alcohol.

☐ I do not smoke.

☐ I manage my stress through exercise, meditation or some other method, and have plenty of time for fun.

☐ I take time off regularly to relax and de-stress.

☐ I like myself and do not judge or criticize myself.

☐ When I look in the mirror, I compliment myself.

Communication

☐ I actively listen to others, asking meaningful questions.

☐ If a miscommunication happens, I deal with it immediately to clear the air.

☐ I do not participate in gossip.

☐ When asked for my opinion, I offer it constructively.

☐ I enjoy encouraging others to be their best.

Final Score

Tally your score (one point for each statement that's true for you) and scroll down to see what your score means: _____

26–30: Congratulations! It appears as if you make living your life purposefully and well a priority and that you maintain a healthy mind-body-spirit connection. What can you do to not only sustain this success but perhaps enhance it for even better health?

21–25: Great! What will it take to achieve an optimal mind-body-spirit connection and wellness on a regular, sustained basis?

16–20: Okay – you have the basics and are ready for more. What support or information do you need to achieve this?

11–15: It seems you are under a lot of stress and resonating at a very low energy. Stress is associated with poor health, anxiety, depression and general unhappiness. Look at the areas in which you scored the lowest. What can you do today to start making living your life well and purposefully a priority? How would it feel to have a partner championing you to success?

Below 11: Thank you for your honesty. This was to encourage you to take a moment to truly look inside yourself and see if you are content with your life. Clearly you have the opportunity to improve your overall health and energetic well-being by making small, sustainable choices that will lead to remarkable, lasting changes. This is YOUR time – long overdue, don't you think?

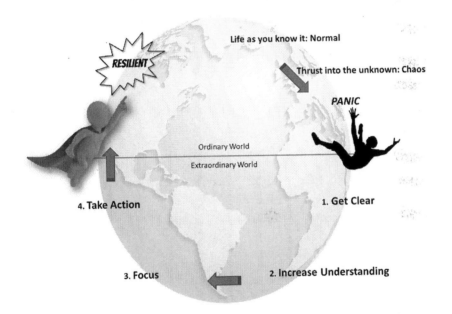

The Ordinary World

But there's a world beyond what we can see and touch, and that world lives by its own laws. What may be impossible in this very ordinary world is very possible there, and sometimes the boundaries between the two worlds disappear, and then who can say what is possible and impossible?
– David Eddings

CHAPTER 1

Don't Panic

Just when the caterpillar thought the
world was over... it became a butterfly.
— Anonymous

How the hell did I get here? The sound of my heartbeat is
deafening as I nervously sit in the stark examination room.
Although the room isn't cold, I am shaking uncontrollably,
silently debating with myself about whether or not I need
to be here. My instincts are telling me to flee, to escape the
imminent danger I believe is about to unfold. It would be
so much easier to simply ignore everything and go home.
Realistically though, I know that's just wishful thinking.

Have you ever had one of those days when everything just
seemed to go wrong and later you were convinced the trajectory
of your life had changed for the worst? Well, I had one of those
days in 2006 when I experienced a sudden physical trauma. At
the time I had absolutely no idea just how far off course life
would take me.

It was 11:20am on April 26th, 2006. While sitting at my desk working on an important proposal, I noticed a tingling sensation in my right hand and a slight loss of vision in my left eye. These are typical warning signs of the onset of a migraine headache for me, so I took a break, got a cup of coffee, took my medication and went back to work. Oddly, the symptoms neither diminished nor increased after an hour, so I took another dose of medicine. It was over the course of the next few days that I realized that the entire right side of my body was numb and I had lost about 50 percent of the vision in my left eye. When I took a long, hard look at myself in the bathroom mirror, while trying not to panic, I said aloud, "Something is dreadfully wrong." Thoughts of a stroke swirled around in my head as my entire body began to tremble.

The following Monday morning I contacted my internist for an appointment. He was out of town and I was scheduled to see another physician in the same office. When I entered the examination room, terrified about what he might find upon examining me, I cut him off at the pass, so to say, and through nonstop chatter explained that I must be stuck in a migraine aura and if he could just get me unstuck, I'd be fine. Not being my regular doctor, he was quick to agree to a cursory checkup. He sent me on my way with a prescription to take my codeine-based migraine medication every four hours for the next three days. If nothing changed or I got worse, I was to call him.

For the next two days I was able to function, but certainly not with all cylinders firing. Thankfully no one at work took much notice of me or how slowly I was moving in my codeine-induced brain fog. But after three days of taking way too much medication without any change in my symptoms, I decided it was time to reach out to my neurologist who treated my migraines. Obviously this was not a typical migraine aura and something really was terribly wrong.

Via an exchange of emails I was able to get in to see my neurologist on Friday before she started her normal schedule for the day. She was late for our appointment and I couldn't relax. Finally she arrived, examined me, asked me a bunch of questions about how I felt and nonchalantly declared that most likely I had had a stroke. Time stopped. *This can't be happening! I'm only forty-four. She may be calm, but I'm fighting the urge to panic.*

She sent me on my way with the non-comforting words: "We'll do a bunch of tests to see where we are. In the meantime, take one aspirin a day and we'll talk on Monday."

I got the required blood tests at the hospital where her office was located. Seven vials of blood were drawn. I heard the clock on the wall ticking loudly. I started shaking again, and the nurse asked in a much too perky voice, "So how are we on this beautiful day?" I burst into tears. *We are terrified.*

Since I couldn't be scheduled for the MRI scanner until later in the afternoon, I went back to work. I had a huge event coming up in a week, and the chaos preceding it was suffocating. With what precious few hours I had, I tried to get something accomplished. Then I left early and found myself being squished like a stuffed sausage into the tiny MRI tube. The nurses were so kind, trying to shift my perspective from "stuffed sausage" to "stuffed cannoli" as they tried not to hurt me while injecting the contrast die. The machine was deafening, even with earplugs. My body continued to tremble, and I knew I was exhausted.

Driving home after the MRI was quite the challenge, as I was distracted and drained from the stress of the day and the week. Within an hour of getting home my neurologist called and said that I had definitely suffered a stroke. I was to continue with the aspirin regimen and get an echocardiogram on Monday. Getting through the weekend seemed insurmountable. Fear was choking me so that I could hardly breathe.

Monday's follow-up echocardiogram showed that I had not had a stroke. In a migraine sufferer who might have experienced a stroke, there should have been a hole in my heart. But my heart was healthy and whole, thank God! My doctor now thought I might have a brain tumor! Sh*t! Considering my potential final days in disbelief, I called for reinforcements, because I was not going down without a fight. And to be honest, at that point in time I felt as if I were truly in the battle of my life.

My reinforcements were my doctor friends with whom I worked. They all came to my aid and reassured me that I did not have a brain tumor, but said that the scans revealed I might have multiple sclerosis. My neurologist thought it was unclear. She kept using the words "maybe," "we think," and "let's wait and see if it happens again."

Wait and see... no way! This is my life we're talking about.

Thankfully there was an MS expert in the Chicagoland area who fit me in for a second opinion in just two weeks (for others there was a minimum four-month wait list). My family went with me to the appointment. After a complete examination and a litany of questions to which it seemed he already knew the answers, he looked directly at me and stated, "My dear, beyond a shadow of a doubt you have multiple sclerosis." I went silent while my mind started screaming. *Did I hear the doctor correctly? Do I really have some illness that will never go away? Can't I be cured with a pill or surgery? How has my life come to this?*

It felt like the universe had sucker-punched me in the gut. The room closed in around me and I began to panic. My heart raced as fearful thoughts spun around in my brain: *I have worked in the business side of health care for over twenty years and live a healthy lifestyle. How did this happen? Why me? Why now? Are you sure?*

As the room closed in I had what felt like an out-of-body experience. Although I was sitting on the examination table, my peripheral vision seemed to have disappeared and it felt like I was floating above myself, barely able to hear anything yet feeling terrified. I focused on my father; he was slumped down in his chair, broken, shocked, his hand covering his face so I couldn't see his fear or tears. Next I saw my mother, her hand over her mouth as if to stop herself from screaming. Far in the distance (but it was actually only across the room) I saw my brother bombarding the doctor with questions. The words "You can die from this" jolted me back to reality. *Time out... I can what?*

As I tuned back in to the conversation I got the doctor to focus his attention back to me. He told me I would not die from MS but that I could die from complications from it. He stressed the necessity of taking good care of myself and prescribed medication. When we left his office everyone was hungry, so we went to the cafeteria for lunch. It seemed like everyone was acting as if nothing had happened. But something had happened, and I couldn't focus on anything else. Life as I knew it was over. Now what?

For the first few days after that I was in disbelief and shock. News of my having MS spread like wildfire. Phone calls, notes and flowers poured in. One would have thought someone had died. I guess in some way I had; or at least my good health had. Although I felt devastated, terrified and angry, my gut instinct told me that everything would work out. Somehow I knew I would get through this life-altering challenge.

In part, I subconsciously knew I could handle this uninvited disruption of my life thanks to the "Panic Game": a game my parents had played with my brothers and me when we were children to teach us how to think strategically and calmly in crisis situations. Playing this game instilled in me a four-step critical-thinking process: 1) Get clear; 2) Increase understanding; 3) Focus; and 4) Take action: I call it the G.I.F.T. My childhood preparation was now being put to the test! Using this instinctive process as a steppingstone, I began the long journey of emerging from the shadows of a devastating diagnosis and being able to say, "I may have MS but MS does not have me."

***

I'm upstairs in the area between my brothers' bedrooms, sitting on the couch with them watching television while playing Mad Libs. Mom and Dad are out and my brothers and I are laughing at the preposterous stories we're creating, when we smell smoke. As it wafts upstairs, my oldest brother begins to investigate. He sees flames at the bottom of the staircase and begins coughing from inhaling the thick smoke. We're trapped on the second floor with no easy means of escape! Oh no, what do we do? We all look at each other and yell, "PANIC!!"

The Panic Game was created by my parents. We would play this around the dinner table a couple of times a month. One of my parents would typically create an emergency-type scenario or a grave situation such as the example I just told of. After they had set the scene they would exclaim "Panic!" and we'd each have to come up with a reasonable solution for the situation without truly panicking. My parents felt very strongly that we needed to be prepared for any situation when home alone so we would know what to do without becoming frozen with fear.

The Panic Game taught me the invaluable skill of thinking on my feet. When in traumatic situations, I keep a level head, assess the situation, come up with possible plans, and then execute what I feel is the best option. Through the years I've been able to master this process so I can do it in a matter of mere seconds. More often than not the outcome is acceptable or better. This is a skill I take for granted until I witness someone else coming apart at the seams when faced with a formidable challenge; then I realize how fortunate I am to have honed this skill when I was young.

Throughout my life I have finagled my way out of harm's way on many occasions, and I guess it can be concluded that the Panic Game was the impetus for my first book, *Live in Wellness Now*, my career, and in general the way my brain functions. Life changes unexpectedly almost every day. Sometimes it does so harshly, as if to slap you, leaving you doubled over in pain and/or shock. Many people in these situations ask, "Why me?" finding themselves on the road to despair or tragedy. Being taught that every problem has a solution and is truly an opportunity to learn in disguise has helped me to never ask, "Why me?" and instead ask, "Why not me?" – the operative response whispered in my brain with an intrinsic, knowing spark of confidence.

I am reminded of a time when I was working at the hospital foundation office and a friend called to tell me that his mother had been admitted to one of our hospitals. He asked if could I go over and "take care of things." Of course I replied affirmatively and went over as quickly as I could. As I approached the room, my friend's wife came running toward me, hysterical. With terror in her eyes she exclaimed, "Is Mom going to die?" I took her by her arms, held her steady, looked directly at her and replied evenly yet authoritatively, "Yes, but not today!" After which I proceeded into the room to assess what was going on between my friend's mother and the hospitalist who was treating her. In a nutshell, I handled the situation by deflating the panic in the room and instilling calm.

There is an old Jewish proverb that says, "Man plans; God laughs." It illustrates how the best laid plans don't always work out regardless of all the planning you do. Imagine not planning at all and simply flying by the seat of your pants. Anything can and probably will happen, chaos ensuing. Planning doesn't necessarily ensure results, but when prepared you are proactive, lessening the severity when adversity knocks on your door. It also absolves you of blame when you think you could have taken better care of yourself. No one is at fault; it just is what it is. The principle I'm highlighting is that planning doesn't necessarily equal prevention, but when prepared for adversity you are better able to cope when and if it does occur.

The Panic Game taught us four simple steps for thinking strategically in a crisis situation such as receiving a diagnosis of a chronic illness. As you become familiar with each and practice them, you will expertly weave them into the fabric of who you are, with each becoming innate to how you behave, cultivating your resilience. As will be discussed in upcoming chapters, how you think affects how you feel, and how you feel affects how you behave. Creating lasting change takes time. Research shows it takes 30 days to change a habit and 90 days to make it stick. Once you form new habits, your actions become automatically proactive instead of reactive.

When I first received my diagnosis it was a struggle emotionally and physically to find my way out of the darkness. Yet had I panicked I might still be lost. By going through each strategic step the Panic Game had taught me I was able to stop, take a breath, calm down and recognize that I had things under control. And if they weren't in control, at least I was in charge of figuring it out. I became my own beacon of light, illuminating the darkness so as to find a pathway out. People say that when faced with adversity you recognize your true strengths, making you stronger. As someone who never really viewed myself as strong, I began to shift my self-perspective. As C. S. Lewis said, "When we lose one blessing, another is often most unexpectedly given in its place." And the blessing I discovered was my own superpower of resilience.

Discovering my resilience allowed me to look at my situation from a different viewpoint, highlighting that it wasn't my fault when I got sick, although it was normal to feel as if it were. Using the Panic Game as a tool for insight into myself, defining my goals, generating new solutions and overcoming physical and emotional obstacles, I was able to fully understand that sometimes bad things just happen. And because I was already in the habit of taking good care of myself physically and emotionally, I was in a strong position to deal with this uninvited intruder.

Let's face it; life is fragile and unpredictable. Yet with the superpower of resilience that resides in you it is possible to rise to every challenge and keep getting back up again. The answer to my question at the beginning of this chapter, "How the hell did I get here," is that it really doesn't matter. What matters are the principles of positive psychology that explain how thoughts affect feelings, which affect behavior; and how I was able to shift my thinking in order to form new habits, setting the foundation of a four-step strategic-thinking process that became woven into the fabric of my well-being. Are you ready to answer the call without panicking when chaos arrives? I promise the journey will be one of growth, support and love.

CHAPTER 2

WHAT IS RESILIENCE?

Our greatest glory is not in never falling,
but in rising every time we fall.
– Confucius

The Latin root of the word *resilient* means "rebound" or "spring back." In her blog that was quoted in an article for the National MS Society's Momentum magazine, Dr. Marla Chalnick, LPC, wrote:

> I often think of my life with MS as a rubber band: When symptoms flare up, I am stretched out of shape and sometimes I think I might snap. Then, with treatment or time, the symptoms dissipate and the rubber band springs back, but never exactly to its original shape. There's a new normal...it took me some time to learn that, and to find my reserves of resilience.[9]

Being resilient is adapting to circumstances through problem-solving and being proactive. It is being flexible on a daily basis – leveraging your strengths, setting healthy boundaries, being grateful, staying positive and being present to the moment. It is living a life that affords you the opportunity to be healthy and happy.

Resilience: Nature or Nurture?

A well-known idiom is, "What doesn't kill you makes you stronger." However, we each react to adversity in different ways, some more readily and with less difficulty than others. Some researchers believe that DNA determines our resilience, while others believe it is a learned response. Whether inherent or learned, there are steps you can take to nurture your resilience that will be discussed throughout *Be Your Own Superhero*. You can think of being resilient as having the ability to bend instead of break when stressed – being more open to and willing to take calculated risks.

A fellow coach and friend recently pointed out to me that I come from a long line of superheroes. I believe that being a resilient superhero is in my DNA, and that this quality was nurtured throughout my upbringing. My parents are remarkable in that they faced many physical and emotional challenges that thrust them into the unknown on multiple occasions, and I watched as they persevered, grew from these experiences and continued to be grateful and benevolent. They are my superheroes and I proudly follow in their footsteps.

More often than not the natural human tendency is to focus on what's wrong, especially when someone is ill or overwhelmed by stress. When you are at a doctor's appointment the first thing you might be asked is "What's wrong?" or "What's bothering you today?" Many people tend to base their regular conversations on complaining and focusing on the negative, feeling victimized by their ill health or limitations. However, research studies reveal that people with chronic disease are often strong, focusing on what is right or well, thus nurturing their resilience.

Resilience is an ability to recover from or adjust easily to misfortune or change. It is the capacity to maintain hope, flexibility, perseverance and courage; the capability to roll with the punches, bounce back and cope in the face of hardship. Resilience is inside all of us. It's the norm, not the exception. Yes, we experience normal and understandable discouragement, anxiety, fear, grief, anger and sadness; those are human emotions. The difference is people with resilience do not become their emotions; they move past them and/ or use them as motivation to empower themselves to combat their challenges. Resilience is more than optimism or a positive attitude; it's having realistic optimism, or the ability to move forward without denial while acknowledging the current situation.

The building blocks of resilience are many: supportive relationships; problem-solving abilities; good communication skills; the ability to cope with or manage negative emotions such as sadness and anger while appreciating positive ones such as joy and happiness; self-efficacy; self-management skills; living mindfully and intentionally – being aware of and in the present moment, and making decisions based on this; and using your strengths in the face of challenges. You do not need all of these to be resilient; possessing only a few is sufficient. And resilience, like a muscle, needs to be exercised.

The challenges and hurdles you overcome in life are, in fact, this exercise.

Resilience is something you have to actively work at and practice. When faced with an illness or other stressor, do you react or respond? When your resilience is weak you can feel threatened. When your resilience is strong you most likely feel challenged in a positive way. As science seeks to answer how much of your resilience comes from your genetics and how much from your life experiences, it is clear that resilience is a work in progress because you are always learning and growing. Recognizing that resilience helps you get through life's tumultuous adventure, you will learn how strong you are as you're tested. If you're living with chronic disease, you're being tested. You are stronger than you realize, empowered by your inner strength of resilience.

When you have a chronic disease you learn to live with something that impacts you silently and/or invisibly. Your challenges may not be obvious to others unless they know you very well. And, realistically, even those who do know you well might not notice. So when you complain people often respond with statements like "Suck it up – you're fine!" or "You look fine so you must be fine." Unfortunately they just don't get how you're feeling and are probably too frightened to want to understand. Being resilient does not mean sucking it up! It means that you take time to educate those who don't understand. If they really don't get it and choose not to take the time to listen, distance yourself from them. Choose relationships that are nurturing and let go of ones that are draining. It's important to remain authentic and honest about how you're feeling, but not to start every conversation with "I don't feel well." If someone always hears that, they may never take you seriously. Keep in mind that resilience ultimately strengthens your relationships.

Even without chronic disease, we all have bad days. We are all human. Oddly enough, though, the most resilient people seem to be those who are facing the toughest challenge of their lives: they are dying. Those who are facing imminent death teach us the most about how to live. However, we are all actually dying every day. That's called aging. And as you age you will be tested. And when tested you will be faced with your own mortality. When this happens, no matter how many times, you deepen your inner superpower of resilience. Overcome adversity; recognize your G.I.F.T.

CHAPTER 3

THRUST INTO THE UNKNOWN

*It's more important to know what sort of a person has a
disease than to know what sort of a disease a person has.*
– Hippocrates

Life is filled with twists and turns that can appear as obstacles
as you traverse each step of your journey. There is always a fork
in the road and you will always have to decide which direction
you think is best. When you ponder your options you probably
think, "What if I can't do it?" Gently question the validity of
your perception of each situation by reaching deep within to
find your genuine truth. Consider shifting your focus from
what you cannot do to what you can; namely, respond with
positivity. With that said, I am reminded of my version of the
"glass half full" analogy. It illustrates how subjective perception
can be and how "we don't see things the way they are; we see
them the way we are," to quote Anais Nin.

Imagine a glass filled to the midpoint with water. Some
people say the glass is half full; others say it is half empty. Most

believe this is analogous to whether you are an optimist or a pessimist. What if I told you it does not matter? It is simply a glass filled halfway with water. What truly matters is how long you have to hold that glass of water. After a few minutes you would think it's no big deal. But if you had to hold that glass for over an hour you might feel differently. Your arm may grow weary and it may even start to shake or become numb. Imagine that glass of water is a metaphor for the obstacles that life has put in your way – your stress. As long as you hold on to that stress, carrying the full weight of its burden, you grow tired and weak. When you learn to let go, shifting your perspective so that you release and overcome the stress, you feel inspired and energized.

The pessimist complains about the wind; the optimist expects it to change; the realist adjusts the sails.
– William Arthur Ward

The path I have followed in life has not exactly been a straight one. It has taken many circuitous routes as I navigated school, family, friends, work, volunteerism and hobbies, always trying to do as I was told so as to please my parents and fit in with my contemporaries, yet never expressing (or ever really knowing) my own ideals. I was and am what one would call a good girl, doing my best to live up to other people's expectations of me regardless of what I wanted – I was (and am) a people-pleaser at the sake of my own happiness. To this day everyone still refers to me as "the good one." This led to a lifetime of feeling like the round peg that so desperately wanted to fit into the square hole yet never could no matter how hard I tried. And as I grew up I focused totally on what I could not do, never realizing how much I could accomplish until recently. "What changed?" you may ask. Let's examine the obstacles or hurdles that have tried to impede my life's journey to see if you relate to any or all of them in some way and to show how they employed my resilience.

Obstacle #1: Being Bullied

Imagine my parents' joy when I was born on their seventh wedding anniversary, my mother marking the occasion by getting drunk on champagne because she and my father were so elated. Growing up in a prominent suburb of Chicago where no one locked their doors was like perpetually living in an episode of *Ozzie & Harriet*. We didn't have everything economically speaking, but we had a home full of love, caring and values. My parents stressed our Judaism, education and unconditional love as the three main thrusts of our lives. Whenever they were angry they always specified they were angry about what we did, not who we were, and they always expected us to do our best at everything we did. For me that was a very high expectation because I lacked the confidence that trying my best would produce "best" results. It didn't always work that way, and I had a difficult time coping with that, not to mention the fact that as an adult I've learned that we all define success in very different terms.

When I was young my father traveled a lot for work and his office was in the city. Mom, on the other hand, was always home – even when I decided to play at a friend's after school. She always made my lunch, drove me back and forth to school in inclement weather and never failed to make me feel better when I was sick or sad. I categorize my parents as such: Mom was the nurturer and Dad was the provider.

By the time I began junior high school my father had begun to do extremely well financially. However, those changes came at a great price. Tragedy struck in 1974 when my father's older brother died of a heart attack in my father's arms on the golf course at the age of 48. My father, who had been so strict and so powerful, woke up to the realization that life was fragile and too short, so we had better make it count. Until that point I think he thought he was immortal, a very common trait of young people. After my uncle's death Dad became more open about his thoughts on philosophy, being contributing members of society, making our mark on the world, living life to its fullest, etc. He also stressed the importance of having a one-year plan, a five-year plan and a 10-year plan so as not to be wasteful with our time. This was all occurring while I was struggling through adolescence – the absolute worst yet very pivotal years of my life.

During my adolescent years it was very hard for me to see life for the positives. I was quiet and shy, which set me up as the target of bullying by the cool kids. Don't ever believe the old adage "Sticks and stones may break your bones, but names can never hurt you." Take it from one who suffered years of torment: names can hurt and leave deeper scars than any stick or stone could ever do. Because I had few friends in high school, I joined our temple youth group in search of socialization. That was my saving grace, for I made many like-minded friends and felt like I belonged somewhere. It was there where I found a safe environment in which to grow up, slowly discovering myself and my spiritualism, and coming into my own as a human being.

In college the bullying continued, much to my chagrin. Here I was, just 18 years old, living away from home for the first time, and a couple of the girls on my dorm floor decided I was an easy mark. Did they just smell weakness on me? I mean, really, how did they know I was weak? Intermittently throughout my college years I was picked on, making me question if there would ever come a time when I would not be a victim of bullying. The only silver lining on this dark cloud was that I fell in love for the first (and maybe only) time.

Obstacle #2: Death

Imagine having a recurring nightmare that a stranger calls in the middle of the night to tell you the man you love has died. Imagine how you would feel, what you might think and how you might react. Unfortunately I did not have to use my imagination.

While watching *Brian's Song* on television (ironically), the phone rang, and when I answered, a strange male voice asked for my mother. When I said she was unavailable (not wanting to say she was, in fact, out of town) the man stated he was a friend of the "F" family and he had something urgent to tell her. I stated I was her daughter and could relay a message. "David, their son, died," the voice said. *What? How? When? Who are you?* I started to tremble, my anger kicking in as a self-defense mechanism as I took the man's name and phone number while yelling at him that I'd call him back. Immediately I dialed the number where my parents were vacationing. In between sobs I barely eked out, "Mom, a man called. David's dead. Did you know?" Almost inaudibly my mother whispered, "Yes, but we wanted to wait until we were home to tell you." My world shattered. All my hopes and dreams vanished. Life would never be the same.

David was the son of my mother's sorority sister. He was my first, and I believe only, true love – my soulmate. When I first met David it wasn't face to face. It was from a photograph his mother shared with me that sparked an instant attraction and feeling of connectedness in me. After we actually met, we continued a long-distance romance throughout my college years. We spoke of marriage when I graduated (he was three years older) and his moving to Chicago. But fate would not permit us to be together. At the age of 23 he was diagnosed with leukemia. And at the age of 26, he died. The circumstances surrounding his death were horrible, and it was the first time in my life I was faced with such utter devastation.

So as not to "ruin" my life, he requested that I not be informed of his illness. Instead he just withdrew from me. I could sense that something was horribly wrong, as he seemed to struggle for words to say to me when we spoke on the telephone, but he would not admit to anything. For a long time I had dreams about a stranger calling to tell me he had died. My dream tragically came true that night in December of 1985.

I was informed of his death after the funeral, at his request, so that I would not sacrifice my life to be by his side as he faded away. Being denied the opportunity to say goodbye and grieve was the most difficult emotional upheaval I have ever experienced. It took a full year of a heavy heart to accept that my destiny would not include him. Oddly enough, it was he who helped me finally accept his death and begin to bounce back from the depths of my despair. In my dreams one night he came to me and we had a long talk. I rested my head on his shoulder and was calmed by his voice. Although I never looked up, in fear he would disappear, I smelled his cologne and snuggled against his favorite red polo shirt. When I awoke the next morning I felt like the weight of the world had been lifted off my shoulders and that I was going to be okay. I have no idea what he said to me, but whatever it was, my subconscious understood and my resilience intensified.

I was now 23 years old and being faced with my mortality for the first time. Life is finite; none of us is getting out of it alive. The unanswerable question is how long we have to live. My five-year and 10-year plans had been obliterated – no more marrying David, having children by the time I was 26 and enjoying a successful full-time career as mother and wife. It was time for the lessons my parents taught me to become much more relevant to my life. I truly wanted to make a difference for the better and leave my mark on this world so that my life would have meaning. The big question was how to accomplish this noble deed. How could I possibly find love again and still achieve my goals of wife and motherhood without David?

Obstacle #3: Divorce

Have you ever been in a relationship in which trust could not exist because the other person was a pathological liar? Imagine over the course of several years allowing yourself to fall in love with a person who appears to love you too. The buildup to your wedding day is filled with excitement, fun and planning for the future. Two days before the wedding you have a fight with your fiancé, but chalk it up to nerves and let it go. On the wedding day you delight in having all the people you love in one room at the same time. You pause to take it all in. It's a fairytale coming to fruition. You say "I do" with tears of joy. The party is a blur of congratulatory hugs and kisses, and when all the commotion dies down it's time to prepare for the first day as Mr. and Mrs.

That first day arrives after a sleepless night with the reality of a long flight and moving halfway across the country to a new home. You're greeted a day later by new in-laws who express their tremendous dislike of you and your behavior. They flatly state that you are only welcome in their home because you are now their son's wife. Your husband does not defend you, and tells you you're on your own now when he leaves for work the next day, meaning you're on your own for life and not just that one day. Fast-forward through three-and-a-half years of constant emotional abuse, and you find yourself confronted with yet another nightmare coming true.

I return home unexpectedly from being out of town. Things don't feel right as I enter the house. I look around, see nothing, and no one is home. I open the refrigerator door to find a can of Diet Dr. Pepper with lipstick on the opening. Neither one of us drinks that brand of soda. Curiosity gets the best of me and I go into my bathroom and closet area. My sink is wet and my toiletries have been used. In the closet, my clothes, especially my nightgowns, are in disarray. Someone has been using my things. I think I'm going to throw up. Disgust boils up inside me until He comes home. When I ask, "Are you having an affair?" He retorts, "How do I know you're not?" The universe slaps me hard in the face and jolts me into reality. Dr. Jekyll, who turned into Mr. Hyde within 24 hours of our getting married, has me trapped in a living hell that I desperately want (and need) to escape. All hope of a happily-ever-after is lost; there is no sense in trying any longer.

After years of torment and neglect, I had lost my self-confidence, my identity, and who I wanted to be. Looking in the mirror I hardly recognized the reflection of the broken woman staring back at me. Thank goodness I still had the morals and values my parents instilled in me. I also had amazing close friends who made me realize that yet again something was terribly wrong and that I had the power to rectify the situation. After a year in marriage counseling I was able to go through the divorce process without feelings of guilt, inadequacy or failure. Going through my divorce helped me rediscover my superpower of resilience. Not only had I run a household for almost four years, but I had moved to a city where I knew no one and had made many friends and established a name for myself in the business community. For the first time I realized I was an independent, resilient person who saw most things in life for the positive – dwelling on the negative only wasted my energy. I also realized that I was a fighter, especially when life got rough, and that no one could knock me down.

Obstacle #4: Diagnosis

Imagine living in Arizona for almost four years, witnessing firsthand numerous women's faces and bodies turning into leathery old boots from sun damage. As an avid sun worshipper I decided to address this fear head-on by seeing a dermatologist annually in the hope of circumventing my skin aging too quickly. Whenever I had a suspicious blemish my doctor and I would negotiate about whether or not it really had to come off.

You see, I did not like the discomfort of the lidocaine injection to numb the area being incised. On one particular office visit my doctor said a spot needed to be removed although it was "probably nothing." It was non-negotiable so I relented. After she put a bandage on the wound, I left her office and went on with my day without much thought.

The next day started with an early meeting, so I arrived at my office later than usual. Oddly there were several messages waiting for me. My voicemail messages were all urgent ones from my dermatologist. She had even left messages on my home machine to no avail. I wondered what could be so important after just one day. I called her office and the nurse stated that she was off for the day and would call me the next day. With a tinge of fear brewing, I insisted someone retrieve my file and read what it said. With much hesitation the nurse put another doctor on the phone who reiterated that I must talk to my doctor about the test results. Furious, I slammed down the phone in frustration. Not more than two minutes later the phone rang and it was my doctor. The spot that had been "probably nothing" was really something. I had a malignant melanoma. I had cancer. Sh*t.

The tumor was thankfully in situ, meaning it was encapsulated. After a plethora of tests it was determined the cancer had not spread and all I needed was surgery. I got off easy, not needing chemotherapy or radiation. I'm very grateful every single day. However, because I did not need treatment other than surgery, most people did not truly believe I had cancer, making it challenging to get the support I desperately needed to cope with the situation. Again I needed to be self-reliant and look deep within to summon my courage and strength.

Obstacle #5: Are you kidding me?

So I was still standing, having emerged from all these major crises. You'd think I would feel stronger, but I didn't. You'd think I would feel alive since I was healthy, but I didn't. I was stuck in my perceptions of a midlife crisis, not having achieved any of my one-year, five-year or 10-year goals by the time I turned 40. At 44 I was on autopilot: successful, but in a career that I really did not enjoy. I say successful because I was a workaholic earning six figures, and at that point in time I measured success by the size of one's paycheck. I was a machine – getting up early, working out, going to work for at least nine hours and returning home at the end of the day only to eat dinner, watch a little television, go to sleep and wake up to repeat the process all over again. My life was one huge load of stress.

Because my work was my highest priority, I waited four entire days before even taking serious notice of the tingling in my hand and the loss of sight in my eye, as described earlier. Have you ever had what people commonly refer to as a "come to Jesus" moment – an epiphany or intuition regarding the truth of a situation no matter how unpleasant? Well, even though I am Jewish, I had one of those several days after ignoring the fact that my entire right side was numb (including the inside of my mouth) and I could barely see out of my left eye. While staring at my reflection in the mirror I said aloud to myself, "Something is dreadfully wrong." My gut knew things were awry and that whatever was going on was definitely not within the realm of normal.

Three weeks, a litany of uncomfortable tests, and far too much speculation later, all I heard was "we think," "it might be," and "let's wait and see if it happens again." *Are you kidding me? I don't want to take uncertain risks with my life!* After seeking out a specialist, the dreaded words were spoken: "You have multiple sclerosis." Sh*t. Here we go again. I was in such shock and disbelief that I had no words.

What Is MS?

According to the National MS Society, MS involves an immune-mediated process in which an abnormal response of the body's immune system is directed against the central nervous system (CNS), which is made up of the brain, spinal cord and optic nerves. Within the CNS, the immune system attacks myelin – the fatty substance that surrounds and insulates nerve fibers, as well as the nerve fibers themselves (think of the insulating coating of a coaxial electrical cable that protects the interior wires). The damaged myelin forms scar tissue (sclerosis), which gives the disease its name. When any part of the myelin sheath or nerve fiber is damaged or destroyed, nerve impulses traveling to and from the brain and spinal cord are distorted or interrupted, producing a wide variety of symptoms. The disease is thought to be triggered in a genetically susceptible individual by a combination of one or more environmental factors. People with MS typically experience one of four disease courses, which can be mild, moderate or severe.

Although MS is different in each person, common symptoms include severe fatigue, difficulty walking, numbness or tingling of extremities, muscle spasms, muscle weakness, dizziness or vertigo, bladder dysfunction, bowel dysfunction, pain, cognitive challenges and clinical depression, to name a few. I experience severe fatigue, numbness or tingling of extremities (at times), tinnitus and dizziness much of the time. I also struggle with cognitive challenges: large chunks of my life seem to have disappeared into oblivion. None of these are incapacitating for me to the level where my daily life is negatively impacted, although in some people they are.

You might relate to some or all of the obstacles I shared and wonder how I deal with them. Like my analogy of the glass half filled with water, if you're the eternal optimist and see it as half full, you believe everything will turn out well. If you're the eternal pessimist and see it as half empty, you worry yourself sick, focusing on negative happenings in the past, thereby preparing for a bad outcome in the future. If you're like me, a realist well-trained by the Panic Game who sees it simply as a glass with water in it that is meant to be drunk or set down, you are resilient, adjusting your sails to the ever-changing winds of life as you continually perfect your course.

CHAPTER 4

DEFINING MOMENTS

We cannot solve our problems with the same thinking
we used when we created them.
— Albert Einstein

Everyday life is filled with stress. Think about how often you feel completely frazzled due to things not going according to plan, especially on a daily or weekly basis. As part of your life journey, an extraordinary stressor or adversity will push you out of your comfort zone and into the unknown. It usually comes without warning, causing you to react instead of respond. For example, when illness strikes you might have no time to prepare for that overwhelming moment when you hear the dreaded words "You have..." and panic involuntarily sets in. It can put a great deal of strain on your relationships, work and body.

In today's hectic world, stress is rampant, causing an increase in disease (and dis-ease), taking a large toll on our physical and emotional health. What can you do to not only prevent falling further down the rabbit hole of despair but to rescue yourself from its depths? When life feels like it is at its worst, you have the opportunity to be at your best. When the proverbial sh*t hits the fan and you start beating yourself up with negative self-talk, you need a virtual *"Moonstruck"* slap-in-the-face, snap-out-of-it moment to help you shift your mindset. Yes, life is hard. Yes, life is stressful. Bad things happen. It is inevitable. So what can you do about it? You need to tap into your superpower of resilience, decreasing your stress and increasing your overall wellness. As Viktor Frankl wrote, "Between a stimulus and response there is a space. In that space is our power to choose our response. In our response lies our growth and our freedom."

The phone rings. I am hesitant to pick it up because I am exhausted. Everyone, and I mean everyone, has been calling. My mother announced to the world that I was diagnosed with MS and everyone is calling to say how sorry they are and to share their stories of illness to compare and wallow together. I am not interested in anyone else. I have to focus solely on me. Yet my energy is sapped; the stress of it all has obliterated me. No one answers the phone, so I do, reluctantly. It's my cousin, who is literally screaming into the phone, "Oh my God, why you? You're the good one!" And without a second's hesitation I whisper, "Because I can handle it." Then I hear what I just said. Wow! This is a huge "aha" moment. Hanging up from that call I have an epiphany that even though I was devastated, exhausted, scared and angry, everything is going to be okay. Instinctively I know I have the courage and resilience to get through this life-altering challenge. It will be some time before I can confidently live well with MS, but I know I will get there.

As you age you have no idea how, or if, your body will betray you. The unknown is a way of life, causing you to embark on the superhero journey over and over. When you have resilience you know you've "got this" no matter the situation. Resilience is the difference between bending and breaking. It's your ability to overcome, especially when faced with adversity such as a devastating diagnosis. It is influenced by many factors, including your current physical and emotional well-being, nutrition and spiritual practices, if any.

When you accept the *call to adventure* when thrust into the unknown by adversity, you experience risk and reward, meeting each test of character and undergoing positive transformation. Although you might not recognize it, you possess some ability or characteristic that makes you extraordinary and will assist you on your journey. My interpretation is that this journey is how you discover the essence of your resilience. And by using this power you shift your mindset from the negative *Why me?* to the positive *Why not me?*

The first step in understanding fear is recognizing the difference between a threat and a challenge. As mentioned previously, this involves your fight or flight response – your brain's physiological reaction to a perceived threat. But there is also human free will, plus the possible belief in a higher power that makes unilateral decisions to punish and/or reward based on behavior. It's imperative to understand that life happens and that how you respond to it is what makes you more or less resilient. Many of us make decisions in a reactive manner rooted in fear. Fear is associated with risk and being anxious about challenging the status quo. How would it feel to instead make decisions in a proactive manner based on choice? I used to avoid risk, which left me stagnant. When I became a risk-taker (calculated risks, of course), life started to unfold in exciting ways. Upon reflection I realized that I equated risk with fear. In the past several years I've learned that F.E.A.R. is just a word – nothing more than False Evidence Appearing Real. It's not based on reality but on the expectation that what occurred in the past with negative results *might* happen again in the present or future. Wow, what a revelation!

But of course the *feeling* of fear is very real. Fear can manifest as elevated blood pressure, a fast pulse or heartbeat, an upset stomach, muscle or joint pain, a migraine headache or any of a number of other symptoms. How can you empower yourself to be fearless in order to avoid tangible symptoms like these? The first thing you can do is acknowledge your fear. It is simply a feeling that is occurring because you are taking a risk, and that is a good thing. Without risk there is no reward; without failure there is no learning. The next things to do are stop for a moment, take a breath and coax yourself to calm down. If you need to, remind yourself it will be okay. Then recognize that within your fear is an opportunity to strengthen your resilience. Finally, be proactive instead of reactive. Ask yourself what steps you can take to achieve a positive outcome. Remember, you have choice! Rid your vocabulary of "should" and "have to," referring to rigid ideas about what you should do or have to do in order to please others. Be confident that you will not make a mistake. Whatever you do, do it with the best intentions. If you try with intention and don't get the outcome you desire, so be it. It doesn't mean it was a mistake. Rid your vocabulary of words with negative connotations. Focus your energy and thoughts on the here and now. Focusing on (or worrying about) the past and the future only fuels your fear. Create a mantra to help you during such times! An example is "I am a risk-taker." Make it a positive mantra and repeat it often. Allow it to shield you like a superhero's cape. Mine is "Remember to breathe and just keep moving; you're okay," so that I continue to move forward and thrive. Using these tips you can decrease stress, thereby achieve greater overall wellness. Fear cannot have any power over you if you don't allow it to. It's time to take risks, move forward, thrive and be fearless!

Once you have your fears under control, reflect on where you've been and where you're going. Have you ever stopped to acknowledge past accomplishments; or, like me, do you only focus on the goals you have not achieved instead of those you have? I often ask myself, "Am I where I want to be in life?" Unfortunately the answer is usually a flat-out, definitive no. However, like a superhero going through their metamorphosis, you realize that if you want to change where you are in life you need to make a shift of consciousness and choose to behave differently by setting intentions – whether daily, weekly, monthly or yearly. An intention is a determination to act in a certain way. This means you *choose* to act differently. Although it's only subtly different from goal-setting, energetically the disparity is tremendous. If you set an intention, you focus your mind on choosing specific outcomes, thereby energetically attracting what you want. Superheroes typically set the intention that their mission is to save the world. How about yours being similar, but including saving yourself in the process?

You're probably wondering how to go about setting an intention, and what type is right for you. Okay – let's circle back to the fear factor in regard to making mistakes. Stop, breathe and acknowledge that you cannot possibly make a mistake if you set an intention with the very best objective in mind. Remember, this is about YOU. We all have the superpower to choose. There is no right or wrong. People set intentions for all sorts of things: family, health, career, etc. It can be specific or broad, and about a tangible thing or an intangible feeling. Whatever in life you want, set the corresponding intention.

Six Steps for Setting Intentions

1. **Set S.M.A.R.T. goals:** Simple, Measurable, Achievable, Realistic and Timely.

2. **Get clear** about what you want. Write it down or say it out loud. Commit to it. It can be as simple or complex as you wish.

3. **Be accountable** to someone else. This will make you more apt to stick to it and not lose confidence.

4. **Keep it simple,** achievable and stimulating so as to keep it doable. Sometimes we jump in full force and set unrealistic expectations. For example, if your intention is to lose weight, expect to lose one or two pounds per week, not 10 pounds in one week – that is not healthy and sets you up for failure.

5. **Create reminders** such as a vision board (a collage of pictures) to manifest your ideal life. Place them in areas you frequent as a constant reminder of the choices you want to make.

6. **Congratulate yourself.** Be sure to acknowledge your efforts when you achieve goals. Too often we let our inner critic degrade what we've accomplished. Quiet that inner critic and celebrate what you've done!

Check in with yourself regularly by taking a few moments out of your hectic schedule each day to ask yourself if the choices you are making align with your desires. Don't let fear of perfection hold you back. Opt for seeking excellence instead, to challenge yourself to do your best without failure. Set intentions that afford you the opportunity for achievement.

Genuine optimism is being aware that problems and obstacles exist and recognizing that there are solutions and workarounds. Grasp that overcoming them won't be easy, and have faith that you can prevail. You know deep in your soul that you will learn and grow. Remember the old adage "What doesn't kill you makes you stronger."

When I was coping with my hurdles, I would have vehemently disagreed with that statement. However, after experiencing my defining moments (one of the most poignant being that of my MS diagnosis), I fervently agree that we learn from our challenges. My "aha" moments defined who I am today by helping me recognize the difference between being threatened and being challenged. This huge shift in perception enabled me to understand my fears and face them head on. And as my thinking shifted I began to understand how to turn my fears into strengths and dig deep inside to cultivate the skills I needed to thrive. Insecurities kept bubbling up as I went through this process, demonstrating my vulnerability, validating the normalcy of these negative emotions and allowing me to acknowledge that although not easy, the struggle was worth the effort. Through adopting the habit of setting intentions regularly, I am better prepared to live fully and completely regardless of any obstacle in my path.

CHAPTER 5

—

A Leap of Faith

When you come to the edge of all the light you have known,
and are about to step out into darkness, faith is knowing
one of two things will happen: there will be something to
stand on, or you will be taught to fly.
— Richard Bach, Jonathan Livingston Seagull

In the last chapter I shared with you my big "aha" moment and that I was now considering a different angle from which to view this health crisis.

I now stand at the precipice of taking that first step in experiencing the first of the four stages one would likely face when receiving devastating news: 1) trauma; 2) grief; 3) acceptance; and 4) thriving. However, in order to take that first step I must escape the bonds of fear and believe in something greater than I think I am at this moment in time. I must find the faith to trust that a virtual net will appear to catch me, or that if I fall I will have the strength to get back up again. Even amid my despair and the shock of mortality slapping me in the face, I must take a leap of faith.

In this chapter, as I share how I summoned the courage to do this, it is my hope that you will find inspiration to discover your own confidence and resilience.

A popular saying is "When one door closes, another opens," and in my opinion, the hallways in between can be a bitch! So there you are, having just received a diagnosis of a chronic health condition, and perhaps feeling like one door has just slammed shut. Let's imagine that as you metaphorically stand in the hallway between the closed and as-yet-to-be-opened doors, a disruption occurs, causing the lights to go out. You're stuck in the pitch black without a flashlight, unable to see anything. Your knee-jerk reaction is to retreat back to the light from where you came. Although it is familiar and you yearn for what was, you cannot realistically turn back the hands of time and undo your diagnosis. In terms of navigating life's journey, this pull to return to what was can be called denial.

At the same time, however, your intuition (your inner sight) speaks to you, encouraging you to move forward into the unknown and reassuring you that all will be as it is meant to be. This can be called resilience. This is your defining moment. How do you want to show up in the world right now? You have choices. You can allow fear to hold you back and keep you stuck in denial, or you can tap into your superpower of resilience and take a leap of faith forward.

Resilience is not just moving into the unknown, but pushing forward regardless of your fear or resistance to change. It is not about giving up or giving in to your circumstances or letting the moment define you. As Helen Keller said, "Life is either a daring adventure or nothing. To keep our faces toward change and behave like free spirits in the presence of fate is strength undefeatable." Let's face it; just like a superhero, you will never know how strong you are until being strong is your only option.

At the moment I heard the dreaded words "You have multiple sclerosis," I remember feeling the room close in around me. All sound faded into the background except for the frantic thoughts swirling around in my brain, the words "You could die from this" jolting me back to reality. I also remember walking out of the doctor's office and my family discussing eating lunch before we headed home, as if nothing had happened; probably too shocked to even acknowledge what we had all just been told. All I could think was *what the hell just happened?*

Fast-forward to the first few days following my definitive diagnosis, and my life was truly a blur. I became trapped in that metaphorical hallway between being in denial and wishing I could turn back the hands of time, and calling on my resilience – knowing that my life had dramatically and permanently changed and that I must find the faith to believe I would be okay.

Between my body being completely worn down from the initial flare-up, and a round of IV and oral steroids to alleviate my first symptoms, I am already in a weakened physical and emotional state. Aside from desperately wanting to hide from reality, my inner critic keeps admonishing me that this is my fault. Remembering that the doctor had connected the dots of my medical history leading to MS, I tell myself that I should never have allowed myself to get sick or I should have known to take better care of myself. None of these thoughts are truthful, but they are all I have. Someone has to be blamed, so why not blame myself?

When you are vulnerable, tired and stressed, as I was, your inner critic (what I call my gremlin) will likely show up and take a leading role, criticizing you, telling you you're not good enough and adding to your stress (and in my case blaming me for causing my disease). Your negative inner voice intensifies your fear, degrading your self-worth and distracting you from your true potential. This, too, is normal, and to quiet the inner critic so you can achieve your potential you have to acknowledge that it's normal and find a way to re-center yourself.

Three Tips to Help Silence Your Inner Critic

1. **Identify the message:** Become aware of what your inner critic is really saying to you and when it is the loudest. Take a moment to consider if the message stems from an experience you had in the past. Be as clear as you can about the source and decide to shift the negative message to a more positive one. To simply ignore the message is not an option.

2. **Acknowledge the message:** Acknowledge how the message has served you in the past. In other words, acknowledge that it has been a loyal guardian, even if misguided. Allow your inner critic to vent, if necessary, before moving on.

3. **Replace the message:** Replace the negative message with a positive one. Like changing the radio station when you don't like a song that is playing, change your internal dialog. For example, change "You're not good enough" to "I've got this and can do this!"

Your inner critic reveals how you feel about yourself. It is not about anyone else's opinion. Look beyond the flaws you think you see into your inner soul and reveal the truly amazing person who is you! I know this is easier said than done. When I first received my diagnosis, I viewed myself as damaged goods, feeling no one would want me because I was broken. It took the encouragement, love and support of my family, friends and medical team to help me silence that gremlin and recognize that being sick was not being broken – that my determined spirit would help me live well and whole even with an illness inside my body.

When trauma or tragedy occurs, often the only thing you can focus on is simply getting through the day. I get that. And if that's the best you can do to start with, then thank yourself for doing that much. You might find yourself focusing on something that seems silly and irrelevant to the important challenges you face and decisions you must make. That's okay, too. It's normal to allow fear to sidetrack reasonable thinking. Have faith that your resilience will prevail. What is not healthy is allowing fear to stop you in your tracks and cause indecision that prevents you from living your life.

Fear is an unpleasant emotion caused by the belief that someone or something is dangerous, a threat, or likely to cause pain. Physically, fear is the distress signal received by the brain that I described in the introduction, called the fight or flight response. With more than 100 billion neurons, the brain is a complex network that manages our bodies, our conscious thoughts and our automatic responses. The fear mechanism is an automatic response that we do not consciously trigger. Without it we could not survive. It keeps us safe. However, as part of human nature we can anticipate fear when we expect something bad to happen. This is a conscious thought over which we have complete control, also known as a *conditioned response*.

While fear is a vital response to physical and emotional danger that helps us protect ourselves from legitimate threats, we often fear situations that we imagine or perceive as threatening and allow them to hold us back. People often fear change, failure or success. Fear of change is the biggest obstacle you can face in life. It is normal to fear change because it is the unknown – that dark hallway between the opened and closed doors. Its pull is so fierce it can paralyze you with self-doubt, anxiety and stress, all of which can lead to disease. If you are wrestling with fear, ask yourself, "How true is this fear? How is it serving me?" This reality check will more often than not help you see clearly that your fears are unfounded and that you are the only one standing in the way of your growth. It's like when I thought I was damaged or broken due to MS; that fear only made me feel worse about myself, which in turn added to my physical distress.

Fear of failure isn't about failing; it's about receiving criticism for the failure and that people's perceptions of you will change. No one likes to be judged, especially for their failures. Ask yourself what my parents always asked me: "What would you do if you knew failure was not an option?" If you cannot fail, then you are free to think about the endless possibilities. Let your fear of criticism motivate you to live in the moment, be present, and not worry about what others or your inner critic might think. Let your fear of failure and criticism motivate you to strengthen your resolve and build confidence. Remember, the only real failure is if you don't take action. If I had allowed fear to prevent me from learning to inject myself with my medication, I would not have slowed the disease progression in my body and thus might not be as healthy today as I am. Given all the information about this medication, I chose to take it in order to help myself, in spite of the potential discomfort it could cause.

Fear of success is actually fear of failure and change in disguise. It's about stepping outside our comfort zone and being filled with anxiety, because no one likes to upset the status quo. As I mentioned earlier, our inner critic likes to remind us that we're not good enough or smart enough so that we stay put in our little boxes. The reality is that we don't fear success so much as we fear being ourselves; and we don't believe we deserve the success we know we can achieve. I challenge you to break old routines and keep up with the physical, social and emotional changes going on around you. (There will be more on this in the next chapter in which you will learn how to bring your gremlin to life as a means of acknowledging and validating these deep-seated fears.)

As you learn to understand the energy behind your resistance to change, use it to your advantage to minimize fear and increase resilience. Let yourself shine and let your greatness spill into the energy of the world. Marianne Williamson said this so elegantly:

> Our deepest fear is not that we are inadequate. Our deepest fear is that we are powerful beyond measure. It is our light, not our darkness, that most frightens us...as we let our own light shine, we unconsciously give other people permission to do the same.

Do you allow fear to hold you back, causing you to remain unfocused? Fear often incapacitates us – even the most successful people. *Marvel Comics* superheroes often find themselves paralyzed by fear when initially confronted by it. Everyone has their own Achilles heel. In your superhero journey this is known as "entering the unknown": a point in the journey when the rules of nature have changed and you are tested against them. To achieve success, shift your thoughts to positive ones, because positive thoughts create positive action. By having faith in yourself, a higher power or both, you come to know and trust your superpower of resilience.

With a diagnosis of MS I certainly was "entering the unknown." I had previously dealt with illnesses that could be cured by either surgery or medication. Never had I been faced with something that was incurable and would never go away. Life felt daunting.

When fear arises in your life journey, begin by identifying the fear and its origins. Then acknowledge the fear and validate its existence. Question how real it is. Finally, replace the message with one that is more positive and powerful. Have patience with yourself and do not lose courage in considering your own imperfections; instead, set about remedying them. Realize you have the power of choice. You can choose to listen to your inner critic, believe it and stay stuck; or, with a little bit of effort, you can try to quiet your negative self-talk. Trust in who you are and recognize that failure does not define you; it proves you made the effort and contributes to your growth.

If you need a little extra assistance to remain focused on the positive, find a talisman that prompts you. For example, when I first received my diagnosis, my personal trainer suggested I buy a piece of jewelry to wear that would serve as a constant reminder of my strength and what I had endured. At first I sloughed off her suggestion. Then one day while browsing at Saks, I saw a ring made of four bands intricately soldered together with several tiny diamonds scattered throughout. It spoke to me, representative of the parts of my life journey coming together in a strong, beautiful fashion, and my spirit soared. I bought it, and to this day every time I wear it I feel empowered.

Breathe to Minimize Anxiety and/or Fear

If buying a piece of jewelry isn't in your budget or sounds silly to you, a simpler method by which to focus on the positive is to practice deep breathing. Often we tend to hold our breath when stressed, or we take shallow, quick breaths, not giving our body and brain adequate oxygen to optimally function. One of my favorite simple breathing exercises to calm you when you feel anxious or stressed is taught by Dr. Andrew Weil, Director of the Arizona Center for Integrative Medicine at the University of Arizona, and a true pioneer in the field of integrative medicine. I have followed him much of my life because he and my Uncle Emil were mycologists together back in the day. All of the information he offers empowers a person to take control of their life and health from an integrative or holistic viewpoint – treating the person, not just the disease. As you practice this exercise, keep in mind that when you feel tension starting to rise up within you, simply bring your attention back to your breath and focus on inhaling and exhaling.

The 4-7-8 (or Relaxing Breath) Exercise from
Dr. Andrew Weil

Sit in a comfortable position with your back straight. Put the tip of your tongue against the roof of your mouth, just behind your upper front teeth, and keep it there through the entire exercise. When you inhale, do so quietly through your nose, and exhale audibly through your mouth. Although challenging at first, you will be able to take slow, deep breaths with practice. This exercise acts as a natural sedative for your nervous system.

- Exhale completely through your mouth, making a whooshing sound.
- Close your mouth and inhale quietly through your nose to a mental count of four.
- Hold your breath for a count of seven.
- Exhale completely through your mouth, making a whooshing sound to a count of eight.
- This is one breath. Now inhale again and repeat the cycle three more times for a total of four breaths. Do not do more than four cycles so as not to become lightheaded.[10]

Without risk there is no reward; without failure there is no learning. You can refuse the call and live in the land of denial, turning away from the adventure for fear of the unknown; or you can blaze your own trail, taking the road less traveled on your superhero journey, beginning with a giant leap of faith. You will either fall or soar. If you fall, get back up, learn from it and try again. And when you do eventually soar, you will experience exhilaration, just as a superhero does when learning to harness their newly discovered superpower. I caution you to not give up too easily. Sometimes you have to be tough, and if you find that impossible, fake it until you make it if necessary, recognizing that "impossible" is simply "I'm possible" with a small shift in perspective.

Now that you know you are, in fact, possible, you are willing to accept the call to adventure and the beginning of change. When you cross the threshold into the new, unknown world of uncertainty, you are empowered based on your ability, not on your disability. Taking this leap of faith, you are becoming the change you wish to be and see in the world.

As I was going through the diagnostic process, one test all the doctors said I needed to endure was a lumbar puncture, or spinal tap as it is more commonly known. As soon as I was told I would need the test, my mind immediately jumped to all the medical television dramas I'd watched and the countless spinal tap procedures that were dramatized. My fight or fight response activated in a flash as I pictured in my mind's eye the pain and anguish these television "patients" had experienced. No one was touching me with that enormously long needle!

Using Dr. Weil's breathing technique to calm myself, I resolved to have the procedure after all, knowing it was imperative, placing my trust in my doctor since she was the expert. As the date of my appointment grew closer my mother and I discussed her holding my hand during the procedure. She kept making halfhearted jokes that as long as she did not faint at the sight of the needle, she'd be okay. Taking serious note of her implied nervousness, I began to consider her emotional well-being and the ill effect it might have on me. To get through this unwelcome event, I needed to be able to look into the eyes of reassurance, not ones that matched or exceeded my own fear. Recognizing I needed to handle this without my mother's help allowed her to remain in the waiting room and not see her child in anguish. Having taken this leap of faith, I probably broke the hand of the young intern who allowed me to hold his during the procedure as I silently cried the entire time out of terror. I'm human. The procedure took less time than expected, and although very uncomfortable, it was not painful. The moral of this story is don't believe everything you see on television or read on the Internet, and once you have made such a decision, trust in your doctor's expertise.

After I received the definitive diagnosis I had to learn to inject myself with medication every other day. A nurse was sent to my house to teach me how to do this. Before she arrived I spent a little time surfing the Internet. To my dismay I found a lot of scary information about the medication, its side effects, and mishaps of self-injecting that made me question whether or not I really could inject myself, let alone tolerate the medication. Once the nurse arrived and we were quietly ensconced in my bedroom, I bombarded her with my extensive list of questions and concerns. When I finally stopped to catch my breath, she calmly put her face up close to mine, stared straight into my eyes and sternly exclaimed, "Stop researching on the Internet!" I was shocked into silence. She went on to explain how misleading the Internet can be and that one must approach it with caution and discernment. She answered my questions about the actual process of taking the medication and explained that my doctor would review the clinical questions I had during my next appointment. Over time I have learned how to use the Internet as a trusted resource because I now know which health sites are reputable.

Had I let fear control me in either of these experiences, I would never have been tested to determine what was wrong with me, nor would I have agreed to take the medication my body desperately needed. As my doctor so eloquently put it, I would have played Russian roulette with my life, which most likely would not have had a favorable outcome. I really had to quiet my mind and reason with myself, determining what was factual and what was nonsensical so I could take the appropriate steps forward with faith in my heart and soul.

When you are in crisis, you experience changes in your life (and body) you never expected. Change is a normal part of life, but when it happens abruptly it can catch you off guard. Imagine you are with a group of people all experiencing crises, and you are all sitting in a circle. Everyone writes their problem on a piece of paper and places it in a pile in the middle, and each person is instructed to select a problem out of the pile. What problem do you choose to take? You take your own problem because it's easier to deal with the familiar. You take ownership of the change that is happening to you, recognizing the opportunity for growth while remaining confident you can handle it. And, with a leap of faith, you embark on the unknown. As the thirteenth-century Persian poet Rumi said, "The wound is where the light enters you."

As you discover your tenacity and courage, gaining faith in yourself, your stress begins to lessen and you embark on a proactive path. Thoughts become clearer, resulting in your ability to make necessary decisions without an abundance of fear attached to them. You might not get rid of all fear, but you will lessen its intensity. And if you find yourself easily distracted by what I like to call "bright shiny object" syndrome – being enticed by more interesting things – bring your attention back to your breath. Literally say out loud to yourself "inhale" and "exhale" as you breathe, changing to silently saying the words as your anxiety subsides.

At this point I bet you're asking yourself, "What if I make the wrong decision?" This is a time to actually investigate where this fear is rooted. Are you fearful of missing out on other options once you've made a decision? Could something from your past that had a disastrous outcome happen again? Has your research on the subject overwhelmed you to the point of being stuck ("analysis paralysis")? It's normal to ask whether you are making the wrong decision. By practicing mindfulness through deep breathing you learn to quiet your mind and hear your intuition speak to you. Intuition is that little voice in your gut that guides you, if you listen. Author and life coach Iyanla Vanzant advised, "The next time you want to know if something is the right thing to do, ask the power within...and pay attention to the response!" This is where your mind and spirit join together to lead you in the direction meant for you. And just like all superheroes, you learn to trust your instincts.

If you are not comfortable trusting your gut (or intuition), ask God/Spirit/Energy for guidance. One way to do this is to begin by setting an intention. As previously mentioned, people set intentions for all sorts of things: career, family, friends, health and so forth. During my first year of living with MS I set the intention that I was determined to overcome all obstacles put in my way so that I could regain some sense of balance in regard to my health. By setting this intention I committed to myself that I would stay the course of treatment even though adjusting to the medication (interferon beta) proved extremely challenging. Even when it seemed my body would never learn to tolerate the medicine, my stubbornness kicked in and I refused to give up. Intentions can be as specific or as broad as you like – for something tangible or for an intangible feeling or emotion. Whatever in life you want, you set the corresponding intention. Outside influences may test you, but if you have faith in yourself and stand strong (or stubborn, as in my case), you will prevail.

An intention is a determination to act in a certain way. When you set an intention, you focus your mind on choosing specific outcomes, thereby energetically attracting what you want. As Buddha said, "All that we are is the result of what we have thought. The mind is everything. What we think we become." Intentions are thoughts directed toward a specific outcome – your consciousness actively shaping your reality. According to Deepak Chopra, "The sages of India observed thousands of years ago that our destiny is ultimately shaped by our deepest intentions and desires." The classic Vedic text known as *The Upanishads* declared, "You are what your deepest desire is. As your desire is, so is your intention. As your intention is, so is your will. As your will is, so is your deed. As your deed is, so is your destiny."

In summary, take a leap of faith and allow life to unfold in exciting ways. The feeling of fear is very real and can manifest as symptoms of disease. Empower yourself to be fearless and avoid those physical ailments.

Seven Tips for Being Fearless

1. Acknowledge your fear. It is simply a feeling that is occurring because you are taking a risk, and that's a good thing. Trust your instinct to guide you appropriately.

2. Take a moment! Stop, breathe and calm down.

3. Within this fear (or adversity), recognize the opportunity or G.I.F.T.

4. Be proactive instead of reactive, asking yourself what steps you can take to achieve a positive outcome. Remember, you have choices. When you catch yourself saying "I should" and "I have to," change your dialog to "I choose to" and "I want to."

5. Remember, you cannot make a mistake; whatever you do, you will do with the best of intentions. If you try and it doesn't work, so be it. Try something else.

6. Focus your energy and thoughts on the here and now. Focusing on past outcomes or worrying about the future only fuels your fear.

7. Create a mantra or get a talisman that is positive. My mantra is "Just keep moving," so that I continue to grow and thrive.

Be cognizant that even superheroes experience fear. And as they strive to better themselves by helping others less fortunate, they take many calculated risks as means to an end for personal growth and solving problems. Remember that fear has no power over you if you do not allow it to. It is time to take risks, cultivate your tenacity, move forward to resilience instead of remaining stuck in denial, and take a leap of faith.

Now that you are ready to take that leap of faith, it's time to implement the lessons of the Panic Game – Get Clear, Increase Understanding, Focus and Take Action so that you can soar. As you tap into your resilience, you are well on your way to becoming your own superhero.

The Extraordinary World

It is the seeker who understands there is more than what meets the eye, who is not afriad and makes the choice to go into the unknown. The process of awaking has begun, the discovery is underway.

— Alan Watts

CHAPTER 6

GET CLEAR

Some are born great, some achieve greatness,
and some have greatness thrust upon them.
— William Shakespeare

Days have gone by and the words "Beyond a shadow of a doubt, you have MS" still reverberate in my mind. My heart feels heavy and I am a bit dazed. A very dear friend from out of town visits to offer love and support. One night we sit alone at the dinner table sharing a bottle of wine. In the stillness of the night we engage in a very raw and honest conversation. With tears welling in my eyes I tell him how broken I feel, questioning whether I could ever be successful in life or be loved by a man considering I am now damaged goods. He assures me that I am nowhere near broken, and he gently helps shift my thinking to the more positive and realistic: that my life is definitely not over, it simply has changed. As I become clearer on the reality of the situation, a small spark ignites within my soul.

Thrust into Chaos

There are four phases of growing from adversity to opportunity. At the beginning of your superhero journey you are thrust into the unknown without warning, entering the first phase: trauma. You experience something deeply upsetting, whether physical or emotional. You probably feel confused, shocked, scared, discouraged and/or hopeless. In my particular case, I felt completely broken, with a strong need to be fixed (and fixed fast!). It was imperative to **Get Clear.**

When something bad happens, you might ask, "Why me?" And when a series of bad things occur in your life, you can feel victimized. You're not alone. It is quite normal to unconsciously see things from a viewpoint of "what's wrong?" and to focus on the negative; that's part of the human condition. But there is a way to avoid the abyss of negativity using a conscious approach to focus on the positive.

When something happens that causes you to exclaim, "Why me?" what if you looked at it from a positive perspective and consciously chose to instead say, "Why me that I get to live a blessed life?" Here's a simple example: A friend of mine recently experienced a horrible accident that could have killed him. Although his injuries were quite severe and he has to endure lengthy surgeries and physical therapy in order to heal, I've never once heard him say "Why me?" from the standpoint of being a victim. Instead he is grateful he thought quickly enough to fall in such a way that saved his life. In essence he says "Why me?" from the perspective of "Why am I so fortunate?"

This brings me to the Law of Attraction, commonly known as a metaphysical belief that like attracts like; that positive and negative thinking bring about positive and negative results, respectively. In his book *Think and Grow Rich*, Napoleon Hill discusses the importance of controlling your thoughts in order to achieve success, the energy that thoughts have, and their ability to attract other thoughts. Simply stated, what you think is what you attract. This is the foundation of tapping into your positivity and resilience.

Do you ever stop thinking? Not really. Even when you're asleep your thoughts continue in the form of dreams. Your subconscious is constant. And your thoughts make you who you are. They determine your ethics, morals and dreams that decide your destiny. How you control your conscious thoughts is the key to living a successful life. We are each a product of our own belief system, and your intuition (or your gut instinct) tells you what to do... if you listen.

What we think determines how we feel, which dictates how we act. Therefore when you think negative thoughts you encourage negative feelings, which make you conduct yourself in an adverse or destructive manner (destructive energy). When you think positive thoughts you awaken positive feelings that lead to constructive or healing actions (restorative energy).

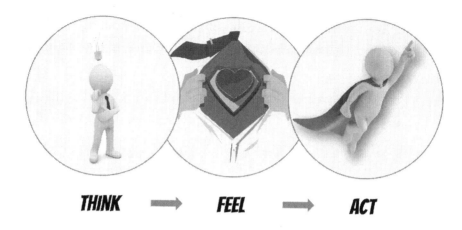

THINK → **FEEL** → **ACT**

To illustrate what this means, here are brief examples from my personal experience:

1. **Destructive thinking:** When I look in the mirror I see a damaged, limited person because I have MS. By thinking this way I feel poorly about myself and have low self-esteem. And because I'm so wrapped up in this self-loathing, I don't eat right, exercise or take care of myself, figuring it doesn't matter how I choose to act because I'm sick. I'm stuck in a downward spiral of negativity.

2. **Restorative thinking:** When I look in the mirror I think I'm strong and congratulate myself for what I've accomplished through healthy eating, exercise, self-care and a positive attitude. By thinking this way I feel proud and have a higher sense of self-esteem. And because I'm filled with positive energy, I make better choices during the day that benefit my healthy living. My focus is on the positive.

As you read each of these examples did you feel your energy shift? If yes, in what way? What you think is really what you attract. You can only feel "less" by thinking you are less. The next time you find yourself thinking negative or destructive thoughts, consider how you can shift them to the positive or restorative, and then pay attention to what happens next. Your mind is a powerful tool.

Struggling with Your Mortality

Upon learning of my MS, I began to question my mortality. The only other time I had really been faced with these thoughts was when David died, because it was so out of the natural order of things. Thinking about my eventual death – now considered to be sooner rather than later – began to consume me. I was distracted by what might be as I aged with MS, a plethora of possible limitations looming in the background. I worried about how my family would cope. And I struggled with the fear of suffering and the pain I might have to endure.

As part of getting clear, I decided to contact my lawyer and put my affairs in order. I updated my will, ensuring everything was organized so that no one would be burdened with undue responsibility in the event of my death. I also signed a medical power of attorney, designating someone I trusted to be my representative in the event I am unable to make or communicate decisions about all aspects of my health care, and specified those choices very clearly with little margin for error. Somehow this act brought me much comfort. In reality I knew I was not going to die anytime soon, but by having my affairs in order and ensuring that everyone pertinent knew about it, I was able to relax and focus on the necessary steps of taking care of myself.

First Steps

I was sitting in the examination room with my head spinning due to the shock of just having received my diagnosis, and the doctor started talking to me about medication. He told me that I must take interferon beta, which is an injectable drug. My eyes got large as the words stumbled out of my mouth: "I have to give myself a shot? Why can't I just take a pill?" My neurologist went on to tell me that the only available disease-modifying treatments for relapsing-remitting MS were injectables, and I had my choice of Betaseron or Rebif. Rebif needs refrigeration but comes premeasured; Betaseron does not need to be refrigerated but I would have to mix it myself. As I stared at him in total bewilderment, he handed me two kits – one for each of the medications – to take home and study before making a decision, although he nudged me in the direction of Betaseron because his team had worked on that particular drug and he felt it was the more reliable.

At this point I was on information overload. Too much information had been thrown at me all at once and I didn't know which choice to make. And frankly I didn't want either option. After all, how on earth was I going to inject myself every day? The thought of it was daunting, making me cringe. Yet when I got home and started looking over the material, it became clear that Betaseron was the option for me because I travel a lot and did not want to have to worry about carrying a cooler with me. I also felt that mixing the medication had to be easy compared to actually injecting it. Once I shared my decision with the doctor's nurse, she arranged for someone from the drug company to come to my home to teach me how to mix and inject the medication. That, unto itself, was a surreal adventure!

The doorbell rings and when I open the door a disheveled-looking woman is standing there with one hand on her forehead and the other holding a bag. She mumbles that she is the Betaseron nurse but has a migraine and needs a glass of water to take her medication. I invite her into our home and my mother gets a glass of water. When she brings it, my mother gives me the look of "OMG, are you sure you want this woman teaching you?" Yes, first impressions are quite indelible and this woman is certainly making one that I'll never forget. After about 20 minutes though, she starts to feel a little better and proceeds with teaching me how to mix and inject the medication. I bombard her with many questions to which her responses are to ask my doctor, she is only here to teach me how to take the Betaseron.

My hands shake tremendously when I put saline into the vile, put together the syringe and inject myself as she had demonstrated. I can feel my heart beating out of my chest. She reminds me to breathe, takes out the real medication and has me mix and take my first dose. I carefully clean the injection site with alcohol, mix the interferon, place the syringe into the auto-injector, try to hold it steady and then depress the trigger. POP! I have to hold everything in place, counting to 10, and then I remove the needle. It burns, but isn't as awful as I expected. I remove the needle and rub the area with a clean cotton ball to distribute the medication from the injection site. "I can do this," I think to myself.

The nurse gathers her things and leaves me with an 800 number to call if I have questions or concerns. I stand at the door watching her go, feeling my head spinning from this all-too-quick lesson.

When I have to take the next dose I am so nervous that I take my mother into the bathroom with me and teach her, just as the nurse taught me, to reinforce in my brain what I had learned. Slowly I go through each step, getting more clear and confident.

After about a month it is as if I have been doing it my entire life. Don't get me wrong; it is still an unpleasant necessity. But I am no longer anxious and feel like I have things under some sense of control.

During a recent visit to my neurologist, he decides in what feels like a matter of mere seconds that I need to switch my MS medication because the old one is no longer effective. Apparently I failed my neurologic exam, plus I've been sick with colds far more often than normal this past year. He puts only one medication option on the table and I'm left with many unanswered questions as he asks me to sit in the waiting area while he completes the data entry for my office visit. As I plop down on a chair in the sun-filled atrium and wait for his nurse to discuss next steps with me, I can feel my heart racing and my eyes begin to tear up. I abruptly stop my imagination from running wild with fear and force myself to take a long, deep, cleansing breath. And then I take another. Okay, I'm slowing down now; my mind is coming back to the present moment and I stop allowing fear to take over. Taking it one step at a time, I get through it.

I grab my phone and Google the new medication. I go directly to the pharmaceutical company's website because they have the most accurate information on the drug. Then I go to the support group on Facebook, skim the comments and jot down questions. The point of doing this is to get clear on what this medication is, what it can do for me and how my body might react to it. The more information I have, the better prepared I will be to make further decisions and tolerate the acclimation process.

The nurse comes to get me with a warm, inviting smile. Immediately I am assured she is in control, understands the situation and knows what to do. We sit and talk for quite some time while she explains in detail the next steps and answers all of my questions. She gives me a brochure to take home along with her email address in case I have more questions or problems. Most important, she assures me that many of their patients who are currently on this medication have done much better than on the one I am currently taking. That is encouraging.

So what is the moral of my story? If you calm yourself at the advent of a crisis situation, become present to the moment, quiet your inner critic and do your homework to learn as much as possible about the basics – namely **Get Clear** about your situation – you will find your resilience bubbling up to help you battle whatever villain is trying to knock you down. Along the way, remember it's okay to ask for help if you need it – to have an extra set of ears at a doctor's appointment, for example. You don't have to sort through the confusion alone.

In summary, when you are thrust into chaos, entering the unknown, whether it be a diagnosis or another traumatic event, recognize feelings of panic bubbling up inside. As you question why this is happening to you, center yourself and become keenly aware that you can handle it. Mourn what was and acknowledge that you have to let it go. You are entering your new normal – learning to cope and recognizing your superpower of resilience. By using positive thinking as a tool to guide your behavior, you are taking the first step to becoming your own superhero.

CHAPTER 7

───

INCREASE UNDERSTANDING

We must be willing to let go of the life we have planned
so as to have the life that is waiting for us.
— Joseph Campbell

Okay, so I have a disease that is chronic and cannot be cured by surgery, chemotherapy, radiation or medication. I am clear on the fact that it can only possibly be slowed down; there is no other option other than to live with it. My instincts kick in and I know I must learn more and do whatever it takes to live my healthiest life. I must take charge, making it my job to take exceptional care of myself for the rest of my life. Of course I'll listen to my physician, but there are numerous other avenues to explore from an integrative approach that address the full range of physical, emotional and spiritual influences that also affect my health that he might not know about. It's time to muster all my strength and venture down that road less traveled.

Now it was time to sort through the chaos, getting my act together while acquiescing to the fact that my normal had abruptly shifted. My doctor at first told me I had had a stroke. The initial tests showed that I had not had a stroke but might have a brain tumor. That morphed into "you might have multiple sclerosis," but honestly it was just guess upon guess, ending with the words "Let's wait and see if it happens again." I found myself so frustrated by this incessant guessing that I persisted and sought out a specialist who offered a concrete diagnosis. Now that I had specific answers to what was going on in my body and brain, no one was offering a way for me to lead a normal (or somewhat normal) life other than by taking pharmacological medication.

As part of your superhero journey, it is time to accept the call to a new adventure and begin the process of transforming your life. In order to do this you have to sort through the chaos that has enveloped this phase of grief, assess where you are in your journey and begin to **Increase Understanding** of the situation. The best way to do this is with my *Wheel of Wellness* tool. Using the Wheel of Wellness affords you the opportunity to check in with how you're feeling emotionally as well as physically at any given moment in time. It is an authentic, holistic snapshot of all the areas of your life, through which you can discover what is true for you, without outside influence, and determine what areas of your life are off balance so you know where to focus your efforts in order to regain stability.

Appelbaum Wheel of Wellness

Keeping in mind that wellness is the coming together of your mind, body and spirit in harmony, begin to set the stage for a prosperous life. There are eight dimensions of wellness, all interacting in a way that contributes to your unique quality of life. They are:

- **Diet:** This refers to the food you actually put in your mouth. I use the term *diet* loosely because it has unfortunately earned a bad rap. People tend the think of *diet* in terms of deprivation in order to lose weight, and even equate it with a four-letter word. But *diet* actually refers to the food and drink you regularly consume for nourishment.

  What is the proper diet for one to have? Our government confuses us with propaganda, first with the Food Pyramid, then a revised version of it called My Plate. Neither shows the vast options for healthy eating for each individual's needs. Both push whatever food the government is currently subsidizing, whether truly healthy or not. So how do you know what you should eat? The simple answer is to talk to your doctor, a registered dietician or a certified nutritionist. They can review your habits and health history, taking into consideration your current health status and goals, and construct an eating plan customized to you. In general it's best to eat real, unprocessed foods with an emphasis on fresh vegetables and fruit; hormone-free, antibiotic-free, organic, lean protein; whole grains; and healthy fats, while limiting sugar, trans fats and alcohol consumption. As you fill out the diet section of the wheel, consider whether or not you eat a well-rounded diet consisting of these options.

- **Weight management:** How much you should weigh is subjective, and I'm not asking you if you *think* you are fat or thin, I'm asking if you truly are or not; whether your weight and *body mass index* are within the appropriate ranges for your gender, height and age. When marking your satisfaction level on the wheel, consider that there is no cookie-cutter, one-size-fits-all weight, and realistically acknowledge whether you are within 10 pounds of what is considered healthy and if you have a positive self-image in terms of your weight. Recent research suggests that the older you are the more you ought to carry an additional 10 pounds to physically protect yourself should you fall seriously ill and loose a tremendous amount of weight.

- **Water intake/hydration:** Do you drink enough water throughout the day? Most Americans are dehydrated because they don't drink enough plain water. Seventy-five percent of your brain and muscles is water. It regulates your body temperature, helps your body absorb nutrients, aids in converting food to energy, removes waste, and more. How do you know if you're properly hydrated? It's simple. If the color of your urine is light or nearly clear, you are properly hydrated. If the color is dark yellow, you need to drink more water. And there is no substitute for plain ol' water.

- **Stress management:** Do you carry the weight of the world on your shoulders, finding yourself tense, holding your breath, grinding your teeth or unable to focus easily; or are you able to relax even under pressure? The longer you hold on to stress, the more of a burden it becomes and the lower the number you should circle on the wheel.

- **Unhealthy habits:** Consider if you smoke, drink excessively, overeat more often than not, don't get enough sleep and/or put everyone else first and forget about or put off self-care.

- **Fun and recreation:** Do you take time to enjoy life and do things that bring you joy? When was the last time you did something *you* wanted to do versus what someone else thought you should do? Do you even know what you like to do for fun, or are you so busy pleasing others you've never taken notice of what brings you joy?

- **Meditation** (or some other spiritual practice): Meditation is a conscious practice using your mind to promote relaxation, develop patience and reduce the destructive emotional effects of everyday life. It facilitates mindful, nonjudgmental awareness of your experiences in the present moment. It helps ground you when you feel like everything is out of control. With practice, you learn to focus your awareness on your breath, a phrase repeated silently or an image in your mind's eye. As you investigate your distractions and notice whether they come from rehashing your past – causing anger or frustration, or worrying about your future – causing anxiety or fear, you learn to focus on becoming mindful instead of having a mind full. Do you spend at least 10 minutes each day in some spiritual practice that promotes mindfulness, gratitude and/or intentional breathing?

- **Exercise:** Studies prove that exercise benefits muscles, bone health and brain health. Exercise can be in various forms: gardening, walking, hiking, jogging, playing sports, swimming, dancing, etc. Do you move for at least 20 or 30 minutes, four to six times a week to elevate your heart rate? Do you participate in weight-bearing exercise at least two times a week for 30 minutes each time to build strong bones and stabilize balance?

In each section of the wheel, circle the number that represents your current level of satisfaction in that area of your life. The higher the number, the more satisfied you are in that area. Be honest and consider where you are now, not where you once were or want to eventually be.

When you have circled a number in each section, connect the circles with a line. Notice what shape the line creates – is it a perfect circle or a distorted version of one? Read on to learn how to find greater balance and understanding of you.

Wheel of Wellness

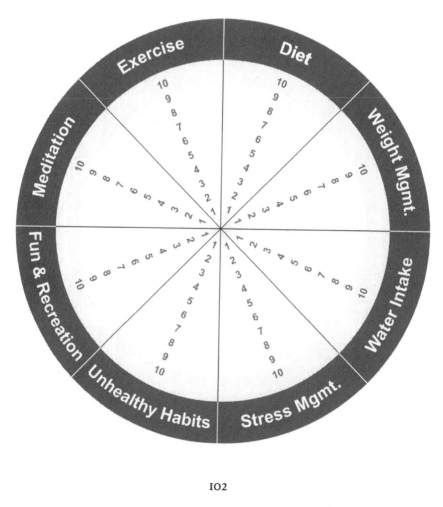

Now that you've completed your wheel and connected the circles, what does the line look like? Chances are you created an imperfect circle. Where the wheel is not round represents disconnect in your life, causing you to experience an uneven, bumpy ride. Think of the wheel as a tire on your car. When it's flat your ride is noisy, very unstable and difficult to control. When the tire is properly inflated your ride is quieter, controlled and effortless. No Wheel of Wellness is ever perfectly round, yet the goal is to strive for it to be as circular and balanced as possible. One client told me her wheel "looked like an old lady bicycle wheel, reflecting my lacking in a few areas but that I nailed others," proving to her that she was consciously aware of a bumpy ride. Another client said she does "not meditate at all but the rest of my wheel is in balance and I'm okay with that." When I completed my wheel after receiving my diagnosis, it looked so out of whack that I never would have been able to control it if it had been an actual wheel or tire on my car. What was your immediate response when you first saw the shape of your wheel? Mine was, "Yikes! I better call for reinforcements by reaching out for help."

Reaching Out for Help: Empathy versus Sympathy

We all need assistance, especially in challenging times. But be careful to choose the right type of help. Initially I reached out to my immediate family and closest friends for moral support and help in understanding what was going on. They are, after all, my lifeline, especially in times of need. At first I had the urge to defend that I was ill, feeling the need to prove just how sick I actually was. When I was young I had a stress-induced Monday-morning stomachache almost every week because I was fearful of going to school and being bullied. My parents thought I was faking it. Yet here I was, actually very sick and definitely not faking it, the reality of which we all had a hard time grasping although my family members were (and continue to be) my rock of stability and support.

It was interesting how some friends responded. There were several who either could not handle that I was ill or could not cope with the fact that they were no longer the center of attention. Either way, they slowly slipped away and the friendships dwindled because I did not have the strength to work at those relationships, which turned out to be acquaintances at best. My true friends were available 24/7 with whatever I needed to get me through, and those relationships were no effort on my behalf to maintain.

Real-life conversations between people with MS on social media tune in to this conundrum of friendships. Many people experience friendships imploding or slipping away, and feel depressed and disappointed.

- "They are scared and don't know what to say or do to help."
- "I found that started before my diagnosis because people just think we are making excuses why we can't do things or cancel at the last minute. It stinks, but I've learned to enjoy my own things in life and if people can't accept me for who I am now, then I won't waste my energy on them."
- "I find that when I laugh others laugh with me; when I cry, I cry alone. So I always try to remember this – people just don't get it until they get it."
- "My diagnosis definitely showed me who was a true friend, but isn't that a good thing? I don't have time for

people now who were not there when I needed them the most. Do what you have to do, for yourself!"

- "I have one friend who has been by my side through thick and thin. I have let her know that I appreciate her so much. We can be out struggling and a stranger will help us out; most people really are kind. I don't want their pity, just their understanding."

Chronic illness will show you two things very clearly:
The amazing compassion of some people you hardly
know at all; and the disgusting selfishness of some
people you thought you knew well.
— Anonymous

I was confronted with the conundrum of wanting family and friends to truly understand how ravaged my body and emotions were, but not wanting them to suffer similarly. When I told people what was wrong with me or how poorly I felt, they just didn't get it. The typical response was "You look fine so you must be fine" or "Oh, I had that same thing and it was _____. Are you sure it's MS and not _____?" When you suffer from an invisible disease, people often think you're faking or that nothing is really wrong. Unlike a cancer patient undergoing chemotherapy who loses their hair, or someone who has broken a limb and wears a cast, a person with a chronic disease might not visibly show symptoms even though their body and spirit struggle with pain or impairment.

What I didn't know at the time was the difference between sympathy and empathy. Many people tend to confuse one for the other, often defaulting to sympathy, which ends up exacerbating the situation instead of supporting it. Miriam Webster defines *sympathy* as "the act or capacity for sharing the painful feelings of another," and *empathy* as "the feeling that you understand and share another person's experiences and emotions: the ability to share someone else's feelings." It is a fine line between the two but there is a huge difference in actuality.

To illustrate my point, imagine you are in a box and you are suffering through some adversity. A family member or friend asks, "Are you okay?" You answer, "No, I'm not," and continue to explain your situation. The sympathetic person will react with, "Oh, that's terrible! I had the same thing happen to me and you know what I did? I ...," making the situation all about them while jumping into the box with you. The empathetic person will respond with, "How you feel is understandable for someone in your situation. What can I do to help?" while keeping the situation about you, standing outside your box and reaching a helping hand inward. And, of course, if someone is apathetic, they won't bother to ask you anything or pay any attention to you at all. That person is definitely not a true friend.

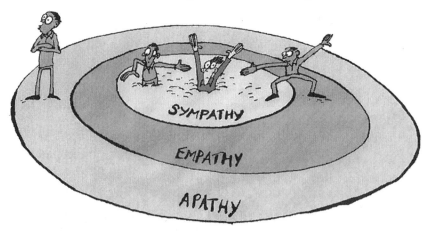

Illustration by Tom Morgan-Jones © Alasdair Cant & Associates
www.cambridgetraining.org

One of my clients who was going through cancer treatment knew she wanted empathy, not sympathy, from her family and friends. She had a friend from whom she had been estranged prior to her getting sick because their relationship was too one-sided. When my client found out she had cancer, her friend wanted back into her life, immediately wanting to be the savior. Recognizing this would be a burden of avoidable stress, my client told her *no*, emphatically. She knew better, and put herself first, seeking out empathetic friends while releasing worry about how others might feel. She knew she had to do this in order to focus all her energy on fighting to beat the cancer.

Keep in mind that it's best to surround yourself with those who express empathy. When you do it inspires love, true caring, and communication that results in genuine understanding of what you are experiencing. As an added bonus, it can also enhance or strengthen those relationships in ways they otherwise might not have been. Allowing people to love and support you affords you the nurturing you need to heal as well as to feel comfortable enough to reach out and gain an increased understanding of your healing.

Learning All You Can

Once enveloped in this nurturing cocoon, I felt supported and therefore capable of focusing on increasing my understanding of MS, how it might affect me physically and emotionally, and what was within my control so I could age as healthfully as possible. I wanted to learn all I could so I became a sponge, absorbing as much information as I could in a very short period of time. I researched online as well as asked questions of my doctors. When researching online,

I went only to reputable websites so as not to muddy the waters with false information (see "Suggested Resources"). To learn what websites were trustworthy, I looked to my physicians and friends in the medical community for direction. I also became acquainted with MS support groups on social media, pharmaceutical websites that provided medications for treating MS, and pertinent newsletters and magazines, as well as the National MS Society and its local Greater Illinois Chapter. If what I discovered included negative rhetoric or caused me anxiety, I ignored it or mentally filed it away to deal with when I was stronger. At this point I figured what I didn't know wouldn't hurt me, and most important, if I didn't know what might happen there was a better chance of it not happening. If I didn't put the thought in my head, then how could it come true? I was putting the power of a positive mental attitude to work. And I learned to adjust, be flexible, go with the flow, trust my gut and remember to breathe. Remember, resilience is bending without breaking – being flexible even in the most tenuous of situations.

CHAPTER 8

FOCUS

Take care of your body. It's the only place you have to live.
— Jim Rohn

After going through hell for almost a year between steroid infusions and adjusting to the interferon-based medication (to which it seemed I was initially allergic), I am exhausted. It has been almost a year since my diagnosis and the person staring back at me in the mirror is unrecognizable. She has become my villain — looking tired, bloated, worn and much older. I'm tired of putting up a brave front; my superhero cape is lying in a crumpled heap on the floor. I'm tired of the interferon wreaking havoc on my body. I'm tired of being treated like I'm sick while at the same time having to put on a brave face. Honestly, I'm so tired I just want to crawl into a hole and hide. I want off this rollercoaster of life, yet know there is no real escape. As I delve further into the unknown, looking deep within my soul, I recognize that hiding is no way to live and not a realistic answer to this situation.

Yet instead of falling down this bottomless rabbit hole of despair, something deep inside reminds me of my childhood training from the Panic Game. I must focus, trust myself and the world around me and start to see this obstacle as an opportunity in disguise. It's time to snap out of it, clear the fog of overwhelm and put myself first on my priority list so I can release stress, gain energy and become the person I want to be versus the person I think I should be.

When you enter this "acceptance" phase – coming to grips with your diagnosis – it's the time to **Focus** on new beginnings. It's the time to discover what you plan to do with your good health and find your purpose and passion for living, while answering the question "How alive am I willing to be?" This is when you begin to emerge from the shadow of adversity as your own superhero, focusing on your mind-body-spirit connection in order to achieve a healthy balance, even with chronic disease.

As I wrote earlier, my professional experience is in health care, on the business side. My medical knowledge is extensive enough to play a doctor on television. Having worked closely with so many physicians, I knew the questions to ask, understood most of the terminology and had developed a practice of looking at the big picture. As my interest in health care grew, I was also exposed to the field of integrative medicine and what that model of health care looks like. Integrative medicine has existed for over 30 years, but has been more readily practiced over the past decade, emphasizing the integration of complementary and alternative medicine approaches with those of traditional medicine. In addition to diagnosis, treatment and prevention of disease, it focuses on the total health of the patient and their overall wellness. Simply put, an integrative approach treats the whole person, not just their disease, transforming the typical health-care model from one based on treating illness to one focused on wellness and disease prevention.

I knew something was terribly wrong when my symptoms began; I just had to muster my courage and decide what to do about it. Once I put up the red flag, letting my neurologist know I was sick and subsequently getting a definitive diagnosis from a specialist, it dawned on me that I wanted a holistic approach to my care, not just medication upon medication, because medicine alone was wreaking havoc on me and I needed a plan to strengthen my body so as to successfully fight this illness. When I reached the one-year mark, I felt like my body was in shambles. I felt like crap, to be honest, and I didn't like it one bit.

My neurologist shrugged his shoulders when I asked what else I could be doing for myself. In his professional opinion all I should be doing was taking my medication. And my current internist, who had just replaced my old one who had retired, was busy with the business responsibilities of his practice and had very limited time to offer me. Trusting my gut, I knew that wasn't enough. And, like when Superman employed Lois Lane and Batman employed Robin as backup in times of need, I put together a team of experts as my personal, professional support system.

To begin, I sought out a doctor who specialized in integrative medicine; who would treat me as a whole person and not just my illness. After asking me a bunch of questions; learning about me as a person, not just a patient; and getting an idea of how I truly felt, he took about eight vials of my blood and ran a thorough check on all my levels – some of which no one had ever measured before. He examined me, watched me walk and administered the usual neurological tests. Then we talked some more.

He told me I needed to shift the way I ate to focus on decreasing my inflammation (a common problem in those who have an autoimmune disease), and that I should see a nutritionist. He told me I needed to shift the way I exercised so as not to overheat (a common problem in those who have MS), and that I should see an exercise physiologist. And he suggested I consider a spiritual practice like meditation to reduce anxiety. As we spoke, we began to create a paradigm for my wellness.

A Successful Personal Wellness Plan

The quality of your wellness today is in direct correlation to the choices you made in the past. And the choices you make today and going forward determine your future wellness. When you choose to plan and then make the conscious choice to act on your plan, you manifest your intentions and live in wellness now. It is also beneficial to have a wellness plan as reinforcement and a method of accountability. Follow this template when writing your personal wellness plan:

1. **Vision:** What is your vision for your wellness? What do you want to do with your good health? Take some time to list what you most desire to achieve and/or experience as a well person.

2. **Intentions:** Pulling from your "vision" list, specify intentions for your personal wellness that you will accomplish over the next 12 months.

3. **Prioritization:** Prioritize the values you will be honoring by bringing your intentions to fruition.

4. **S.M.A.R.T. Plan (Specific, Measurable, Achievable, Realistic and Timely):** What goals and objectives must be achieved in order to fulfill your intentions without compromising your values?

5. **Action Plan:** Create a prioritized list of action-oriented tasks to complete your intentions for the year. Break them down into daily, weekly, monthly, quarterly and yearly tasks.

6. **Commitment:** Get clear about your plan. Commit to it by putting it in writing. Or create a vision board (like I did) and place it where you see it every day so your subconscious can absorb the messages you want to receive.

Creating a Vision Board

A vision board, often referred to as a dream board, helps you harness the power of your intentions and visualize them so you can achieve your dreams, as in the Law of Attraction. To create a vision board, first become present to the moment through a mindfulness activity such as meditation, yoga or even doing a walking meditation through a labyrinth if you live near one. Once you become present, start thinking about who you want to be and how you want to show up in the world right now. Next create an atmosphere conducive to creativity and introspection. Maybe put on your favorite music in the background or light a fragrant candle to inspire you, and prepare a large workspace so you can spread out while you design your vision board.

Have a wide variety of magazines on hand to peruse. Cut or rip out any photo, graphic, saying, etc. that speaks to you or mirrors your intentions. Once you have a stack, arrange them on a piece of poster board (I used an 8" x 14" piece, but feel free to make a larger one if you wish). Once you have an idea of the format, glue the pictures in place with a glue stick. Use markers to add words, symbols or pictures where you feel compelled to do so. If you prefer, there are also books and apps you can purchase to create a digital vision board. Take your time – a few hours at least. Take note of your thoughts as your subconscious mind invites the change you want to experience. Allow yourself to dream big, letting your light shine bright as you release negative thoughts and embrace positive self-discovery.

Place your vision board where you will see it often, perhaps the bathroom mirror, the refrigerator, a bulletin board or the cover of your personal journal or notebook. Or scan it and save it to your computer as wallpaper or a screen saver. The key is to place it where it will remind you to *think* the thoughts you need to think in order to *attract* what you desire in your life. And when you begin to notice the positive changes occurring in your life, celebrate you, your achievements and your vision board.

Below is my vision board as an example. The messages it conveys to keep my subconscious laser-focused are about staying positive, not giving up, believing in the power of my dreams of becoming a well-known author and speaker, that I am surrounded by love and that life is filled with endless opportunity.

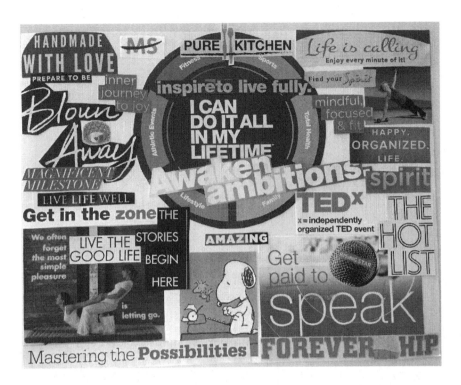

Wellness is the foundation of a successful life. We often hear, "If you don't have your health, nothing else matters." Truer words were never spoken. I know from firsthand experience that not living true to yourself can make you sick. Seeking validation from others can be exhausting and confusing. Striking a mind-body-spirit balance can seem impossible. On the surface your life might seem enviable, yet the pain inside is slowly eating away at your individuality. Not knowing what is true or authentic for you and putting on a façade in order to be successful in the eyes of others are draining. Maybe on some level you know how you "should" act but never seem to follow through for one reason or another. You're not alone. There is a reason you feel the way you do. You might not be able to see it yet, but by focusing on creating a paradigm for your wellness you gain a greater awareness of self; discover your superpower of resilience in order to unleash your true purpose; see clearly what choices you have; and feel empowered, energized and directed toward a more purposeful and successful existence. It is time to embrace change, thrive in forward movement and move on to the next step: **Take Action.**

CHAPTER 9

─────

Take Action

Health is a vehicle, not a destination.
— Joshua Rosenthal

After getting clear, increasing my understanding, and focusing, the reality of my new normal begins to sink in. I begin to view this reality without judgment. I see that although things have changed, I am still quite capable. It's time to take action, putting to work everything I am learning and shifting my lifestyle to a holistic one. It's time to really get my life in order and figure out what I want to do with my good health, once achieved, while honoring my body in addition to my superpower of resilience. By taking action I can begin to accept my new normal with excitement and move forward with living a well life, recognizing that I am fully capable of meeting each test of character as I experience risk and reward.

My father always taught us not to sweat the small stuff in life and to focus on what's important. But how do you discern what is the small stuff and what is important? There's a well-known story that illustrates how to determine what's important in life for you:

A teacher walks into her classroom and sets a glass jar on a table. Without words, she places large rocks into the jar until no more can fit. She asks the class if the jar is full and they reply, "Yes." She questions their response, pulls out a bunch of small pebbles and adds them to the jar while shaking it a bit so they fill in the spaces between the larger rocks. Again she asks, "Is the jar full?" The class quickly agrees it is. She then adds a scoop of sand to the jar, filling the spaces between the rocks and the pebbles while asking again, "Is the jar full?" This time many in the class are not sure how to answer. As they look on with interest piqued, the teacher takes a pitcher of water and fills the jar to the brim while making the observation, "If this jar represents your life, what does this experiment show you?"

One perspective is that no matter how busy you are, you can always do more; typical of people on overload, trying to do it all. Another interpretation is to look at the large rocks as representing the big things in your life, what you really value (such as family, health, dreams); the pebbles as the things in life that give it meaning (such as your work, home, friendships); and the sand and water as the "small stuff" that fills your time (such as watching television and running errands).

The teacher now says, "Imagine if I had started filling the jar with the sand or the pebbles?"

Starting with the big things, I initially took action to put my affairs in order. Yes, the doctor said I would not die from MS, yet added that I could, eventually, from complications due to the disease's effects on my body. And since I am a planner (and worrier) by nature, it put my mind at ease to get everything organized. I put together a financial plan so as not to have any outstanding obligations that might prove a hardship in the future, and I began to loosen the purse strings a little bit. Focusing on saving for the future but not being so cheap as to put off living for today (I am a huge saver, sometimes at the expense of living my life enjoyably) afforded me the freedom to splurge on what would bring me joy. For example, knowing that my future of being able to wear high heels was no longer guaranteed, I purchased an exquisite pair of high-heeled black suede boots with crystal studs up each side. They were a tremendous indulgence, and I figured I was worth it! Every time I wear them, I feel energized and super empowered.

A big thing you might consider is writing a "legacy letter" to your family and closest friends that expresses what matters most to you in life. We don't often get to speak frankly with loved ones in this fashion because it makes people feel uncomfortable. People don't generally like to talk about their true, deep feelings about illness and death, or to reflect philosophically on their life's purpose. Sometimes it's best to put these thoughts on paper in the format of a letter that you know will be read at some point in time, thereby leaving nothing unsaid. Things you might put in the letter include asking for forgiveness if you feel you've hurt someone, thanking a person for being in your life and the role they played in it, telling someone how proud you are of them, or simply expressing your acceptance of your illness (or situation) and how you hope others, too, will find a way to cope. You are in essence sharing your resilience with your loved ones, helping them discover their own.

It's Time to Thrive

You typically play many roles in life: daughter/son, sister/ brother, mother/father, spouse, employee, boss, caregiver, nurturer, etc. You do everything for everyone. Extraordinary demands are repeatedly placed on you at home and at work. You are already a superhero in many ways. Only one thing is lacking: because you were taught to put everyone else first, self-care is something you forgo, sometimes by choice and other times by necessity. You might consider it selfish to think about you first, but it's necessary; because what good are you to anyone else when you're completely exhausted and worn down?

Wellness, as defined earlier, is "an active process through which people become aware of, and make choices towards, a more successful existence." It's not just the absence of disease, it's about balance. When you're playing superhero to everyone in your life, it's easy to lose your balance. Very few take time out for themselves amid a life full of taking care of others. Sound familiar? Remember the Wheel of Wellness? Is your wheel round or quite distorted?

As you take this final step to becoming your own superhero, you enter the "thriving" phase, in which you **Take Action.** Here you discover new beginnings, such as adjusting to and accepting a new normal after a diagnosis, and finding your meaningful purpose in life. Robin Roberts of *ABC News* often touts this wise quote by her mother: "Make your mess your message." You can do this by cultivating relationships that nurture, deciding what to do with your good health and living a healthy life with chronic disease rather than being defined by it.

Most people seek wellness in order to be happy. Perhaps the reverse is actually true: seek happiness and you will achieve wellness. Happiness comes from within. It is found by shifting to mindfulness from having a mind full. It is about accepting yourself, flaws and all, and sharing your gifts with the world in order to make it a better place. It is about pursuing your own excellence, not some unobtainable idea of perfection. Many people have written about the top habits of successful people. One of the main themes in such books is to focus on right now. Don't worry about yesterday, focusing on regret; and don't allow anxiety to minimize your forward momentum in the future. Be present; live in the now.

How to Live in the Now: Mindfulness

Mindfulness is the current buzzword that's everywhere, and there is a subtle nuance but significant difference between being mindful and having a mind full. *The Huffington Post*, *Science*, *The Wall Street Journal* and *Psychology Today*, to name a few, have all published several articles on mindfulness. There are apps, magazines and pages of search results on Google all relating to mindfulness. So what's the big deal about it? Mindfulness helps keep cognition strong and optimistic, especially in someone like me who has MS and is post-menopausal.

Cognition refers to your memory and ability to think. It involves the way you concentrate, multitask, learn, remember, understand, recognize, and problem-solve. We are all unique, and our distinctive cognitive skills allow us to function in everyday life no matter what that looks like to us. My cognition is affected in a multitude of ways, the severity depending on whether I'm having an MS exacerbation, experiencing an abnormally fatiguing day, or all is status quo. For example, on most normal days I have trouble with the following:

- Remembering names
- Remembering prior conversations
- Delays in brain processing (exhibited by difficulty with word retrieval, or "tip of the tongue" syndrome)

However, when I am severely fatigued, I also have difficulty with:

- Concentration
- Coordination (I develop a bad case of the "dropsies")
- Excessive fatigue or drowsiness
- Vertigo or dizziness

My symptoms are not uncommon, and whether you have an illness like MS or are enduring the "brain fog" of menopause or simple aging, you might experience challenges with your attention span, multitasking, learning or decision-making, to name a few. I find my cognitive limitations to be quite frustrating, which is normal. When I try to explain to people why I can't remember something, they often get upset or impatient with me, implying that I use my MS and/or my age as an excuse or crutch, when in fact they are legitimate reasons. Again, it's the "You don't look sick so you must be fine" attitude. Thankfully most days I'm living and aging well, even though most days I experience cognitive limitations.

According to the National MS Society, research shows that approximately half of all the people living with MS have, or will develop, problems with their cognition, yet only 5 to 10 percent of those people experience problems severe enough to interfere with everyday activities. Changes in cognition can be caused by several different factors including medications, depression, stress, fatigue, drug and/or alcohol abuse and sleep disorders. When your body is in a weakened state, at times your brain is, too. A neurologist can either test you or refer you to someone who does the testing to possibly pinpoint the cause(s) and offer treatment options.

According to the National Institutes of Health, "In many chronic illnesses, long-term pro-inflammatory responses, medication toxicities, and/or cellular damage from the disease process itself can impact the integrity and function of the brain...contributing to brain dysfunction."[11] Deficits in memory and attention combined with emotional distress can directly impact a person's capacity to manage their chronic illness due to reduced brain function and reduced motivation for self-management. According to the *Journal of Post-Acute and Long-Term Care Medicine* there is increasing evidence that the older you are, if you have a chronic disease such as congestive heart failure or atrial fibrillation, the more it is strongly associated with cognitive decline. "There is increased evidence showing that other chronic diseases like heart disease, stroke and diabetes, as well as risk factors including depression, obesity and sleep, are associated with cognitive decline. If left unchecked, these chronic diseases can increase a person's risk of developing dementia."[12]

In regard to brain fog caused by menopause, much research has been done with few definitive answers. Cognitive issues related to menopause are most likely part of the natural aging process. However, it is important to note anything unusual, as it may be a sign of something more severe to discuss with your physician. Pharmacological treatment options are available and should be discussed with your doctor if your cognitive limitations negatively impact your daily life. You might also want to explore whether or not you have a sleep disorder. Severe fatigue and sleep deprivation are often correlated to cognitive deficits.

Being mindful is a non-pharmaceutical method for combating cognitive deficits. Some strategies I use that you might find helpful include:*

- Making lists and keeping them in prominent places
- Using Post-it® notes as reminders (I have them all over the house)
- Dividing large, complex tasks into smaller, simpler tasks
- Eating nutritious "brain foods" like nuts, berries and wild-caught or organic fish
- Playing brain fitness games such as Lumosity on your smartphone or computer
- Exercising 20 to 30 minutes per day (any type of movement or exercise has been shown to improve brain health)
- Meditating to become present to the moment, increase gray matter and activate synaptic pathways in your brain, promoting neuroplasticity
- Focusing on the task at hand and investigating distractions in order to minimize them, while avoiding multitasking

These are NOT replacements for treatment prescribed by your physician.

To determine whether your mind is full or you are being mindful, pay attention and refocus your mind when daydreaming. Be aware of and investigate any distractions. When distracted or daydreaming, are your thoughts coming from your past, based in anger or frustration; or are they about the future, filled with anxiety or fear? Remember, what happened in the past is not likely to happen again, and the future is completely unpredictable unless you've discovered the all-coveted crystal ball. And if you have found that, we need to talk!

Many people who have impaired cognition function effectively in their daily lives as I do. If you feel you are not functioning effectively, consult your physician to see what can be done about it. Otherwise, live the best life you possibly can and try a few of the strategies I listed above to be more mindful. Help your body and your brain be resilient so you can live well as you age.

The Importance of Gratitude

Another valuable component of thriving and taking action is developing an attitude of gratitude. Research has found that the value of gratitude includes good health by playing a significant role in your sense of well-being. In 1986 Dr. David Snowdon, one of the world's leading experts on Alzheimer's disease, embarked on a revolutionary scientific study on aging involving a unique population of 678 Catholic sisters. In his book *Aging with Grace: What the Nun Study Teaches Us about Leading Longer, Healthier, and More Meaningful Lives,* Dr. Snowdon inspires readers with stories of these remarkable women whose dedication to giving back and being grateful may hold the key to all of us living healthier, longer lives. One significant finding of his research was that a good attitude, faith and gratitude, along with a sense of community, can add years to your life.

When you practice gratitude, you have a greater sense of self-worth, confidence, strength and energy. This is accompanied by a tendency to experience less stress and being more directed to what you want in life. Interestingly enough, it has also been discovered that embracing gratitude in your personal life promotes reciprocal gratitude in others. This exemplifies *like energy* attracting and encouraging *like energy*, especially that which is positive and healing. It also suggests that you can influence those around you simply by being thankful. For example, take note if someone's energy shifts to the more positive the next time you remember to say "Thank you," even in response to the smallest of actions.

You might ask, "Sometimes it's challenging to be grateful, especially when someone keeps pushing my buttons; do you have any suggestions to help?" In fact I do. First, a person can only "push your buttons" if you have buttons to push. So try to defuse any sensitivity you have that you know someone might attack. For example, stop reacting when your reaction is exactly what the other person is after. Instead, take a breath, measure the value of reacting against that of responding or doing nothing, and choose to not react. Sometimes I find that silently repeating a mantra to myself over and over helps keep me calm, centered and focused.

Here are some of my favorite mantras that I use during those very real and very difficult times to help me stay focused on what's important to me:

- I am grateful for my health. It's more valuable than money or superficial things representative of wealth.

- I am grateful for my family and friends. Their support of me knows no end and is my foundation of being.

- I am thankful that I remain faithful and that my life is filled with purpose, whether apparent or not, and that it is filled with meaning.

- Even when someone does not understand me, I am grateful that my intentions truly are rooted in love regardless of whether others recognize that fact or not.

Gratitude unlocks the fullness of life. It turns what we have
into enough, and more. It turns denial into acceptance, chaos
to order, confusion to clarity.
— Melody Beattie

Community and Socialization

Another way to build your resilience is through socialization and a sense of community. Dr. David Spiegel, Director of the Center on Stress and Health and Professor in the School of Medicine, Associate Chair, Stanford University School of Medicine – Psychiatry and Behavioral Sciences, gave a lecture on the mind-body connection. He said that one of the best things a woman can do for her health is to have strong relationships with her girlfriends, while for a man one of the best things is to be married. Women support one another on a primal, emotional level, creating more serotonin in their brains to combat depression and engender a sense of well-being. Women share from the depths of their souls and talk about practically everything. Men share activities, such as sports, exercising not only their bodies but their sense of camaraderie, too.[13]

Being with like-minded individuals and being part of a community help you feel stronger and more positive. You're no longer facing adversity alone; there are others walking similar paths with whom to share ideas and vent frustrations, minimizing feelings of isolation. Think of when our country faced one of its worst disasters on September 11th, 2001. Although at odds over politics, we came together in the face of tragedy, heroically coming to each other's aid. Although this is an extreme example, the primary focus became preserving human well-being, which is built on a foundation of resilience. According to the National MS Society, a survey of more than 1,500 people with MS and other chronic diseases revealed that "resilience...is linked to satisfaction with social roles (such as work and family responsibilities) and quality of life."[14] Human beings want to engage with other human beings; it's part of who we are and helps us be our best selves. Ways to engage with others and be part of a community, even if you are ill or unable to expend much physical energy, include:

- Volunteer: helping others fills you with a sense of satisfaction and pride and brings you into the community
- Join a support group: reaching out to others who are in similar situations or like-minded helps you not feel isolated or alone
- Go to church or synagogue: joining in worship offers you a sense of community, faith and friendship
- Get involved online (if you can't go out) with groups or in conversations that interest you

Making Bold Choices

In order to move forward, sometimes you need to ask for assistance or for something you need. If you don't ask, you don't get. As simple as that sounds, it isn't. Many people have trouble asking for things they want or need, held back by fear or worry. As a child I rarely asked for anything because I was always fearful I would be denied, made fun of, or worse, get what I asked for and then change my mind. Growing up, maturing, and experiencing life have taken me out of my fear-filled, shy inner shell and opened me up to being a more outgoing, risk-taking person. I'm not so much of a risk-taker that I jeopardize my safety, but I choose to make bold choices whenever things need a little shaking up to keep life interesting, or when I know I need help reaching a desired goal.

Whenever I appear to be on a track I don't feel comfortable about, I think of what I can do to get on a more palatable path and encourage myself to take a leap of faith. What's the worst that'll happen? If I fall and go splat (like I have so many times before), I'll get up, lick my wounds and start again. Not a big deal. Now for the caveat – I only behave this way regarding work-related actions. I'm still overly cautious, shy and introverted when it comes to my personal life. I guess all the bullying when I was growing up scarred me more than I realize. You might even say it is my kryptonite.

A perfect example of this is several years ago when I met a woman through social media who posted that personnel from the Bravo network came to her to put together a cast of women who would be ideal for a new reality television show. It would be a motivating, empowering and uplifting show about how women can really kick ass – her words, not mine. When I walked in the door for the interview she was yelling at her sons while the other candidates congregated in the kitchen, chaos ensuing. The women were dressed in stilettos and slinky, skimpy, very revealing dresses, and wearing too much makeup, and I felt completely out of place; my kryptonite kicking in as my self-confidence waned.

As the hostess sat me in front of her computer for the interview, there were a lot of distractions, making it difficult to focus, causing my confidence to wane even further. As the questions came, I instinctively called on my superpowers of courage, confidence and resilience. When I shared my journey with MS, the whole interview shifted. Quietly the interviewer said her brother had had MS for over 20 years and wasn't doing well. She was extremely frustrated with his lack of motivation to be proactive. We discussed best practices for taking care of yourself when you have a chronic disease, and I ended up coaching her for 15 minutes on how to deal with her frustrations of not being able to change him, only herself. Looking back, I believe divine intervention put me at that Bravo interview in order to make a positive difference in someone's life, helping her discover her power of resilience. And by helping a stranger in need, I also practiced deflecting my kryptonite, which solidified my taking action through practicing gratitude and mindfulness and silencing my inner critic; that is to say, I flexed my resilience muscle big time, and it felt great!

Implementing G.I.F.T.
Four Real-Life Stories of Resilience

Remember that life is not measured by the number of breaths
we take, but by the moments that take our breath away!
– Vicki Corona

Now you know the four-step strategic-thinking process of
G.I.F.T. for discovering your resilience. You've transformed from
feeling broken to being empowered; from being disabled to
being enabled. Although you might still be hesitant, wondering
if this process really works, by taking these superhero action
steps you have become your own superhero. And in case you
are still not quite able to see this in yourself, here are several
real-life examples of people other than me dealing with chronic
disease who, through implementing lessons from the G.I.F.T.
process to discover their superpower of resilience, are being
proactive toward achieving wellness.

CHAPTER 10

BRAIN HEALTH AND AGING

Our minds influence the key activity of the brain, which then influences everything; perception, cognition, thoughts and feelings, personal relationships; they're all a projection of you.
— *Deepak Chopra*

The Story of a Loving Spouse and Caregiver for Someone with Alzheimer's

Several years ago two Baby Boomers, a 55-plus-year-old woman and her husband, faced a life-altering crisis. He received a diagnosis of early-onset Alzheimer's, which rocked the entire family to its core and thrust them into an unknown world overflowing with panic and apprehension. As defined by the Alzheimer's Association, Alzheimer's, a progressive disease that is not a normal part of aging, "is a type of dementia that causes problems with memory, thinking and behavior. Symptoms usually develop slowly and get worse over time, becoming severe enough to interfere with daily tasks."[15] Her husband is one of approximately 200,000 Americans under the age of 65 who have received a diagnosis of early-onset Alzheimer's. This devastating news affected everyone differently: her husband was in denial; she, the spouse and primary caregiver, was devastated and grief-stricken; and her son was very sad and anxious about what it meant, yet remained positive there would be a cure by the time things turned for the worse.

Learning to live with this disease and fighting to stave off progression became the entire family's journey to discovering their superpower of resilience. Putting the G.I.F.T. process to work, they continued with their normal exercise and nutrition plan, but they modified them to accommodate her husband's limitations. For example, he had been a devoted yogi for over 25 years, and his practice has continued six days per week; it has become his lifeline. She is positive that this is what has slowed the progression of his Alzheimer's. He added walking several miles a week, and meditation, and he eats a healthy, balanced diet of organic chicken, fish, vegetables and salads. Because life is short and meant to be enjoyed, he still splurges occasionally on ice cream, which he loves so much! He is a musician, and they found a wonderful music-oriented organization nearby that he attends three times a week, keeping his brain stimulated in various ways. They found a routine that works for them; one that is vital for maintaining balance. Establishing a routine is actually beneficial for everyone dealing with chronic disease.

With her family under constant stress, this woman needed to find a way to take care of herself so she wouldn't get sick herself from combatting the constant exhaustion and sadness of dealing with this seemingly impossible situation. Her superhero strategies include keeping a large supply of tissues in her car for crying while driving. Since she is in constant grief she allows herself some time every day to feel her sadness and grief before going about her work day. She tries to walk every day, and uses a convenient phone app for guided meditation. These strategies allow for validation of strong emotions as well as their release, even if for only a little while. She tries to get a manicure/pedicure and foot massage once a week to care for her body, and attends a weekly therapy group. Staying busy helps, although she's become a bit of a workaholic, causing her to never feel 100 percent relaxed or rested anymore, proving that being your own superhero takes constant effort. She works at staying in the moment and not getting ahead of herself, but it is not easy. Recently she hired someone to be a companion for her husband a couple days a week for a few hours in the hope that it will de-stress her a little and be fun for her husband – a win-win.

In regard to patient advocacy, she goes with her husband to all of his medical appointments, although there's not much to the appointments; usually a simple checkup biannually accompanied by a blood test. Her husband has been on the same medications for a long time and adheres to his physicians' instructions. He prefers not to go to his neurologist because she just tests him, something with which he has a hard time and finds humiliating. When he told the neurologist he felt it was a waste of time to come in, she responded, "I have to agree with you. There's really nothing we can do for you under the circumstances, other than to monitor you. As long as you're doing well, there is no need to come in." So he has never gone back and it's been several years. (Unfortunately medicine is still a practice. And although a physician may not be able to "do anything more for you," it is still beneficial to get checked at least once a year to ensure nothing has occurred that your untrained eye can't detect. It is always better to be proactive than reactive.)

As a result of nurturing his body, mind and spirit to the best of his ability, rarely does he feel ill. His wife can't remember the last time he had a cold. He is very healthy and in wonderful shape. He looks much younger than his age, and they attribute that to his regular exercise and spirituality practice. There are no specific doctor's orders other than to enjoy every moment, and he does. His wife has noticed that if he gets over-tired he experiences a bit more anxiety, but he's able to calm himself down. He rarely complains, lives in the moment and sees the best in everyone and everything. That's one of the positives of the disease: typical human filters disappear and you live life in the present moment, filled with gratitude and abundance. Although he has definitely declined, he still moves forward. Their motto is "Keep on keeping on."

Brain Facts

In order to discuss brain health and the role it plays in discovering your superpower of resilience, you first need to get acquainted with your brain. The human brain weighs about three to four pounds, consists of 80 percent water and 20 to 25 percent oxygen/glycogen, contains over 100 billion neurons, and is the consistency of soft butter. As previously stated, once thought to be finite or static, the brain is now known to be malleable, leading to the understanding of brain plasticity. Neuroplasticity is the brain's ability to reorganize itself by forming new neural connections that allow neurons (nerve cells) in the brain to compensate for injury or disease. When new neurons are generated it is called neurogenesis. In order to maintain cognitive function as you age, you need something called *brain reserve*, which is, in essence, your brain's resilience.

Let's Talk Brain Health

According to Richard Carmona, MD, MPH, FACS, 17th Surgeon General of the United States, in his book *30 Days to a Better Brain*, although we are living longer we are not necessarily living younger. He espouses keeping our brains healthy to support our active bodies, and discusses avoiding stress, anxiety and depression because they play major roles in keeping our brains healthy. This can be accomplished by changing our behavior to be more resilient, which is important to long-term brain health. Negative self-talk – the gremlin, or false thinking – adds to stress, which leads to oxidative stress, which leads to diminished brain health. By using *reframing* we can shift our thinking to feel more present in the moment, less fearful and more optimistic, which stimulates brain health and leads to substantial changes in behavior.

Your mind has the capacity to grow stronger as you mature. Research reveals positive effects from living in a supportive community. Socialization and spiritual faith can create brain reserve. The story at the beginning of this chapter confirms this. We're an aging population, fearful of cognitive decline, and we're living longer and are in need of strong, agile minds to keep up with and maintain our strong bodies. Through simple lifestyle alterations you can slow down degeneration and even enhance cognitive function. When you think, feel and act healthy, your brain stays healthy. And when your brain is healthy, you are able to think, feel and act healthy. It's a symbiotic relationship between your body and your brain. There are core competencies for health – skills and approaches to improve your overall wellness, including brain health. These include exercise, nutrition, stress reduction, sleep, challenging yourself and mindfulness; very similar to the core elements that impact your overall life balance.

Exercising is an excellent way to improve your memory and protect your brain cells. Through exercise such as walking several miles a week like the man with Alzheimer's, a secreted protein called brain-derived neurotrophic factor (BDNF) acts on certain neurons of the central nervous system and the peripheral nervous system, helping to support the survival of existing neurons and encouraging the growth and differentiation of new neurons and synapses. In the brain BDNF is active in areas vital to learning, memory and higher thinking, which are important for long-term memory. To keep it simple, I like to think of exercise as aerobics for your brain, or *neurobics*. Exercise is not just about going to the gym. It can be dancing, walking or playing sports, as long as you find a way to move that gets your heart rate up. Be sure to include weight or resistance training because that is beneficial for bone health, especially as you age. If you are concerned about how much and what type of exercise to do, ask your doctor or seek out a specialist who will direct you according to what is right for your individual body.

You've heard of the *standard American diet*... it is not exactly what one would call healthy since it contains things like fast food and processed foods (hence its acronym, SAD). It's best to focus on a balanced diet of not only healthy foods, but also of healthy relationships, physical activity and spirituality. Proper nutrition includes not only *what* you eat but also *why* you eat. Eating a diet rich in antioxidants that inhibit oxidative stress in your body's cells contributes to better brain health. Eating foods that are not processed and are made with real, natural ingredients is best for your overall well-being. Learn how to read nutrition labels, eat primarily foods with ingredients you can pronounce, and shop the perimeter of the store where most of the unprocessed foods are on display. Choose organic, lean protein; foods with no artificial sweeteners (they actually make you hungrier and possibly cause disease); foods containing antioxidants like dark berries (your cells die when exposed to oxygen, and antioxidants combat that process to keep cells healthy and vibrant from the inside out); and drink plenty of plain water because hydration is super important in keeping your cells and mind healthy as you age. An added benefit of good hydration is that it keeps wrinkles at bay, too! A few foods that are healthy for your brain include blueberries; blackberries; spinach; garlic; turmeric; dark, leafy greens; red wine (in moderation); nuts; green tea; fatty fish (wild caught or organic); olive oil; and dark chocolate (70 percent cacao or higher) – my favorite!

Stress also plays a major role in brain health. According to Dr. Gary Small in his book *2 Weeks to a Younger Brain*:

Stress contributes to other psychological manifestations that are not so obvious, including anger, confusion, depression, impatience, irritability, and memory loss. Stress also leads to physical symptoms like pain, appetite change, fatigue, headache, and insomnia. People who suffer from excess stress are more likely to develop heart disease, high blood pressure and diabetes.[16]

And when any of those diseases are present, you are apt to develop neurologic impairments that can lead to disease like Alzheimer's.

Adequate sleep also helps minimize stress and improve brain health. While you sleep your body heals itself through cell regeneration, and neuroplasticity takes place. If getting enough sleep is challenging for you, try napping. Naps, as needed, are a good option, as they can give you that second wind you might need to get through the day. Just closing your eyes and resting for five or 10 minutes is helpful if taking a full-fledged nap is impractical; although a 20-minute nap will keep you in the lightest stage of non-REM sleep, making it easier for you to get up and go after your snooze.

Another way to reduce stress and maximize brain health is to challenge yourself with a puzzle, a balancing feat or a new way to do something. Challenge yourself by brushing your teeth while standing on one foot, using your less dominant hand to write or taking a different route to a regular destination. Try to keep yourself on your toes, break routines and keep your brain aware and present to the moment.

Mindfulness, mental stimulation and a meditation or spirituality practice are also fundamental to building brain reserve. Studies such as one conducted at UCLA suggest that "meditating for years thickens the brain (in a good way) and strengthens the connections between brain cells...further proof of the brain's neuroplasticity."[17]

Part of maintaining or improving brain health through meditation is cultivating an awareness of the present moment. As previously mentioned, you can do this by investigating whether your distractions during meditation emanate from the past, indicating anger or frustration; or stem from the future, indicating worry or fear. A loose definition of the term *worry* is "planning for a negative future." Think about it: As you worry, you increase your stress and negative thinking, which negatively impact your brain health. If you shift your thinking to the positive you promote neuroplasticity, decrease stress and increase your energy, thereby helping stave off age-related disease. Meditating is a great way to become present.

Meditate to Become Centered and Present to the Moment

One way to cope with the initial trauma of chronic disease is to mourn or grieve what you have lost. Just as when someone you love dies, you have to acknowledge what you've lost in order to move on. Validate your feelings of sadness; you are human, and those feelings are natural. You will miss what once was. However, the key is not to wallow in this emotional state too long, as demonstrated in the story above about the man who has Alzheimer's disease.

Now is the time to tap into your spiritual beliefs and feel supported as you grieve the loss of your good health and begin to accept your new normal: life with a chronic disease. You can, of course, develop your own meditation practice. The one I suggest below is based on my studies of healing prayer and the books *10% Happier* by Dan Harris and *Meditations from the Mat* by Rolf Gates and Katrina Kenison. Doing this type of meditation helps you take that necessary breath amid all the chaos, get clear and focus on the present to become mindful in the decisions you need to make for your next steps.

Find a comfortable position, whether sitting or lying down, in a place void of distractions. You can be on the floor, in bed, on a chair, or on a cushion. Just make sure your back is straight, your limbs are relaxed and you are not straining your neck or head.

Gently inhale through your nose, feeling the cool air tickle your nostrils as your lungs and belly expand. Gently hold your breath for a moment, and as you exhale through your mouth, feel the warmth on your tongue and lips. Find a gentle rhythm of inhaling and exhaling, never straining, simply following your breath. If your mind starts to wander, bring your attention back to your breath and say to yourself "inhale" and "exhale" as you breathe in and out. Actually feel yourself breathing. Your breath should be calm and measured.

Forgive yourself if your mind continues to try to wander. This is normal. Recognize it and bring your attention back to your breath. Sit or lie quietly, just breathing, focusing solely on your breath for 10 minutes. When finished, open your eyes, slowly start to move your hands and feet and slowly get up. Take a mental inventory to see if you feel any differently. I bet you feel much calmer and centered.

If your interest is piqued and you want to learn more about meditation, there are countless CDs and books that can guide you through creating a personalized practice.

In a recent webinar I guided attendees through this meditation to become centered. One woman stated that her experience with the meditation was "fabulous" because she was listening while snowshoeing on a ski hill in the mountains and had stopped, lain down in the snow and stared up into the sun-filled sky. She felt she was nourishing her body while also nourishing her brain. The combined activities created a unique and incredible experience, leaving her exhilarated, and she did breathing exercises on the biggest mountain peak over and over again.

I'm Present. Now What?

Perhaps you have some deep-seated feelings that need to be acknowledged and validated in order for you to move on to the next phase. This is where you get another glimpse of your superpower of resilience. Resilience is important, especially to someone living with chronic disease, because every day you have no idea how (or if) your body will betray you. The unknown is a way of life. When you have resilience, your inner strength, you know you've got this no matter the situation. You learn how to let go of the things you cannot control and focus on the positives and on things you can control, enjoying being present to your journey.

As a brief review, resilience is influenced by many factors such as your current health status, how that affects your physical and emotional energy, nutrition (what you eat and why you eat), spiritual practices (if any) and whether your attitude is one of gratitude or ingratitude. I define resilience as being able to cope or deal with a situation and being able to bend, not break, so you don't fall completely apart when bad things happen. It is the foundation of transformation. It is the ability to recognize the power deep within you that can guide you to the destiny of your choosing.

> *Your body hears everything your mind says.*
> – *Naomi Judd*

As you take steps forward toward transformation, your inner critic or gremlin sometimes appears, knocking you off your confidence pedestal, causing you to feel trepidation and possibly take a few steps backward. This is so normal and so annoying at the same time! In order to quiet your gremlin, try this exercise I learned from reading Rick Carson's book, *Taming Your Gremlin*: Make a physical representation of your gremlin. *Hmmm... what does my inner critic look like?* I had never given it any thought even though I consistently listened to a relentless stream of negative self-talk. I couldn't come up with any great ideas, ironically causing my gremlin to yell at me about how pathetic I was.

But while standing in line at the pharmacy one day, I saw a shelf filled with stuffed animals that were quite odd looking. I asked the sales associate what they were and she replied, "Uglydoll. They are all the rage with the kids!" Uglydoll®... I let that sink in... then it hit me – *that's it! Uglydoll is my gremlin!* It came in various colors and I chose orange because that is the color representing the National MS Society.

Okay, so now I owned an orange Uglydoll. Now what? As I held it in my hands and took several deep breaths, allowing myself to relax into the feel of it, it came to me to write all of my negative thoughts on its backside, or a$$. Makes sense, right? I began with, "You are" and continued with the words that loomed in my subconscious on a never-ending audible loop: "ugly," "fat," "diseased," "lonely," "tired," "limited," "damaged" and "unsure." As easy as it was to write all of these negative feelings, it was super difficult to acknowledge them and let their weight be felt by my emotional heart. I cried. And I cried some more.

Then I asked myself from what was my gremlin protecting me and what dreams or goals was it preventing me from achieving. I had to really focus on whether its message was really true or it was speaking falsely to hold me back. As I pondered the true purpose of my self-criticism I began to understand that I was allowing fear and poor self-esteem to hold me back from taking risks and truly living life to the fullest. I recognized how harshly I was treating myself, and as my resilience kicked in I started to feel stronger and more positive.

With a deep, cleansing breath, focusing on what I wanted my life to really look like, I turned it over to the front side and wrote, "I AM" at the top. "I AM" is a phrase used in healing prayer that indicates you are one with God/Spirit/Energy. Anything you put after "I AM" shapes your reality. I slowly and deliberately wrote words beneath "I AM" that reflected all the positive emotions or characteristics I wanted to be or feel: the authentic messages I wanted and needed to hear. Naturally this part wasn't so easy, and took much more effort to envision.

These are the words I eventually selected to put after "I AM": "well," "a fighter," "strong," "beautiful," "empowered," "smart," "growing," "movement," "full of life," "positive" and "caring."

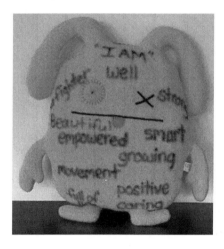 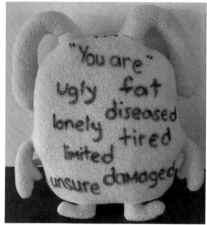

Whenever I start feeling down or weak, or my gremlin starts yelling at me, I pick up my Uglydoll (which I keep conveniently nearby on my office bookshelf) and turn it so I can read its backside: all the obnoxious things it tells me, like a broken tape recorder looping over and over again. I read the words aloud, slowly, allowing myself to feel them at my core and telling myself it's okay to feel this way, temporarily. Then I turn it over and confidently state aloud all of those affirmative words, silencing the negativity and filling myself with positivity and hope.

Whatever your gremlin is like, you might have to fake it until you make it sometimes to really accept the positive affirmations as your truth. Yet with practice you can transform to really believing and embodying them. Be gentle, patient and forgiving with yourself, and allow real change to occur.

CHAPTER 11

―――――

AN INTEGRATIVE APPROACH

*The doctor of the future will no longer treat the
human frame with drugs, but rather will cure
and prevent disease with nutrition.*
– Thomas Edison

An Epiphany at 50 – A Gen X Woman's Story of Living with Lupus

I actually feel quite naive when I look back on my health and wellness. I started having significant joint pain at 15 years old and was misdiagnosed and undiagnosed until my 30th birthday. By the time I had two babies and was in my late twenties, I was in almost constant and excruciating pain. When I eventually received my diagnosis of systemic lupus, I could not lift a glass to my mouth. I read anything I could get my hands on and went to numerous doctors in search of the best treatment. The overwhelming response was meds, meds and more meds. That set me on my journey in constant search for the perfect cocktail. I had the best care that money could buy.

I knew that lupus was an autoimmune disease and that it caused inflammation, but I had no idea that my lifestyle or the foods I ate could contribute to how my lupus was behaving. I quickly discovered that I need more rest than the average person, and my stress needs to be kept at a minimum. But all things considered, I thought I was living a healthy lifestyle. However, as I approached 50 my mindset changed. I wasn't thinking of my lupus as much as preventing heart disease, cancer and Alzheimer's. Fifty was a WOW moment for me, not to mention having five masses removed from my bladder, colon, intestines and ovaries. They were all benign, but this was a huge wake-up call. And welcome to instant menopause due to the hysterectomy!

Recently my dear friend introduced me to a new nutrition plan called Whole30. The rules include eating moderate amounts of meat, seafood and eggs; lots of vegetables; some fruit; plenty of natural fats; and herbs, spices and seasonings. The focus is on eating foods with very few ingredients, all pronounceable, and whole, unprocessed foods with no added ingredients. My friend has also been treated for various maladies over the years, and on this eating plan she feels better than ever.

I was skeptical, but I bought the corresponding book. The plan cuts out all foods for 30-plus days that can cause inflammation. After at least 30 days, restricted foods are reintroduced to the diet one at a time. If no inflammation symptoms appear, then great! If the reintroduced foods cause problems, you eliminate them.

Potentially inflammatory foods are sugars, alcohol, all grains (including corn), beans, dairy, soy, carrageenan, MSG and sulfites. I realized that sugar is in literally everything. I have always been a label reader and a "healthy" eater, but this plan takes it to another level.

I decided that I could do anything for 30 days. Eating lean meats, vegetables and fruit was easy. Not drinking wine was quite hard. Without even appreciating what was happening, I realized after a little over a week that I felt fabulous. After three weeks of eliminating all inflammatory foods, I felt like a teenager! I had boundless energy, my brain felt clear and I was happier. Yes, happier! I have been adhering to the non-inflammatory way of eating for three months now, occasionally reintroducing a potential inflammatory food, and I am always disappointed when I do. Even a small amount of grains, beans, sugar or alcohol causes me to feel sluggish and achy. My advice to everyone is to get the yucky out of your diet! Eat clean and real. If you can't pronounce it, don't eat it.

I have always been a busy and active person, but I am now making more of an effort to focus on exercise. I do anything and everything: swim, bike, run, row and lift weights. I mix it up to keep it interesting. Now that my lupus pain and fatigue are at a minimum, I have the energy to actually go to the gym. I used to need a nap in the middle of the day but now that is a foreign concept. With a clear mind, I have a vision board, I am starting a business with my husband and I am looking for ways to volunteer.

I know that I am not getting younger, but I am going to feel the best I can at 50 and at every age thereafter! I can't control everything, but I have complete control over how I treat the body and mind the good Lord gave me!

Create a Paradigm for Your Wellness

Imagine transforming your health-care model from treating illness to treating wellness, with a focus on prevention, like the above woman did when she turned 50! By concentrating on your health care and not your sick care, you make yourself a healthier patient and can save money and undo stress in the long run. And by taking an integrative or holistic approach, you are respecting your individuality and what wellness means to you biologically.

Everyone has a different interpretation of wellness. Wellness is individual; we are each unique, physically and emotionally. But we need help creating our personal wellness objectives and understanding how to achieve them. Being told "Go home and exercise" means nothing without personalization. We are all living longer and want to live full, active lives – without pills, with an understanding of what's causing an issue and with strategies for addressing change through behavior modification instead of pharmaceuticals. You might think you're doing something healthy when in fact, without realizing it, you're doing something that's not healthy for you at all.

By creating a paradigm for your wellness, you are setting up goals and a system of accountability to those goals. You are also shifting your mindset, realizing that doctors are not just for prescriptions; they are for wellness checks and understanding underlying conditions so you can take individualized right steps to change your behavior. Quick fixes are rarely successful, and pills do not cure; they only mask symptoms. You must get to the root of the underlying cause of your distress. And you must look at your whole person, not just your disease.

Annual screenings, although important, are not considered preventative medicine. Taking care of yourself before you get sick is. Do you ever wonder why some people get sick all the time and others don't? Those who stay well understand how to support themselves and their immune system, manage their stress, eat healthy, exercise, etc. They understand that excessive stress, poor nutrition and lack of exercise are the main culprits of inflammation, leading to getting sick often, because they suppress the immune system.

A Sample List of Anti-Inflammatory Foods

Almonds	Artichokes	Asparagus	Avocados	Basil
Bell peppers	Bok choy	Brussels sprouts	Cabbage	Carrots
Cauliflower	Celery	Cherries	Chives	Cilantro
Coconut	Cucumbers	Endives	Fresh peas	Garlic
Ginger	Jicama	Kale	Leaks	Lemons
Lentils	Limes	Onions	Oregano	Pumpkin
Red beets	Red cabbage	Sea veggies	Sesame seeds	Spelt
Spinach	Sprouted seeds	Squash	Sweet potatoes	Tomatoes

As you age, your body produces fewer vitamins and less nutritional support (such as vitamin D3 and calcium). Supplementation might be necessary, and it's best to consult your physician or find a certified nutritionist to help you choose the right supplements for you. Look to food-based vitamins because they are more natural sources and therefore more likely to be absorbed by your body than pills and powders. For example, to get adequate calcium in my diet, I choose to eat a plethora of dark, leafy greens high in calcium such as kale, spinach and broccoli. But when it came to vitamin D3, I was severely deficient and needed to take a supplement to increase my vitamin D to an acceptable level. Through testing I also discovered that my body does not methylate properly, so I need to supplement my low vitamin B level with a methylated version. Vitamins and nutrients play a role in your wellness by supporting your immune system. Through a simple blood test your doctor can evaluate the best way for you to optimize them.

Another simple habit of preventative care is to wash your hands and not depend on hand sanitizer all the time. Wash thoroughly, singing the entire "Happy Birthday" song to yourself for the proper length of time. If you do this often throughout the day, especially whenever you enter your home after being in public places, you will minimize the spread of germs and illness.

Finally, let's address sleep. As a society we are sleep-deprived, which affects stress levels, mental health and our immune systems. Unfortunately numerous studies have found that there's no catching up on sleep. Once lost, your body cannot catch up, and your immune system and metabolism are depressed.

To figure out how much sleep you need as well as how much sleep you are actually getting, keep a diary for two weeks, noting the number of hours you sleep each night. Track how you feel and note the hours of sleep you got on those days you feel really great and the ones when you don't. Also track what you ate or drank to see if it correlates to the amount of sleep you get and how you feel the next day. Take note of when your mind is most active, and ask yourself if you're under a lot of stress. Examine what's going on in your life, how it affects you as an individual and how you feel, emotionally and physically. This record will help you see patterns, and when you understand them you will gravitate to what you did on the days you felt better. You are providing yourself positive behavioral change in a simple manner and connecting your mind, body and spirit. If you track excessive sleep deficits and cannot figure out what's wrong, consult your doctor or a sleep specialist to ensure that something more serious isn't an underlying cause of your lack of sleep.

The human body is an incredible, fine-tuned machine. Find what you like in regard to exercise, nutrition and a spirituality practice, keeping it simple, real and fun. I like to follow the 80/20 rule: behave 80 percent of the time and splurge 20 percent of the time so you achieve a realistic balance. And like the woman with lupus, be mindful that moderation is the key to almost everything in life, and that when you fuel your machine properly it keeps working efficiently. Once you get into good habits, when you do misbehave your body won't like it.

You're only human, and not all areas of your life can work optimally at any given moment in time. In order to manage what's not working, the key is prevention. To practice prevention, get a baseline understanding of who you are as an individual. Measure it using data points and manage it by noting what made you feel better or worse. Document everything in a log or journal and discuss it with your health-care practitioner. Personal awareness and accountability are the most important components in creating a healthy paradigm for your wellness. When you approach it from an integrative perspective, you use the best medicine from any number of environments including pharmaceutical, technical and medical, combining them with a holistic, mind-body-spirit approach. No one situation fits all people. Treat yourself as an individual, using an integration of multiple modalities to create positive results in the least amount of time. Create awareness; create change.

CHAPTER 12

———

Exercise/Movement

Fitness — if it came in a bottle,
everybody would have a great body.
— Cher

A Young Millennial Woman Living Well with MS

A vibrant 27-year-old woman lives with multiple sclerosis. She lives an extremely active and stressful life that includes work, family and friends. The tools she implements to take action in order to maintain health while staving off disease progression as much as possible include paying attention to her exercise, quantity of sleep, and nutrition.

Exercise is her go-to technique in her healthy lifestyle toolkit. She tries to work out a minimum of 30 minutes each day (which admittedly doesn't always happen). In the summer months when the humidity is at its highest level, it is extremely difficult for her to exert a lot of energy because of how terrible humidity makes her body feel due to the fatigue, pain and inflammation it causes. She tries to vary her routine, mixing it up between running, weightlifting and cardiovascular (cardio) exercise such as Zumba™, kickboxing, using a StairMaster® or using an elliptical training machine. She is an avid runner and also walks and practices yoga, with the goal of moving as much as possible.

She tries to get at least seven hours of sleep per night. That is not always possible or easy, she notes, but a goal nonetheless. Fatigue is a typical side-effect of MS, one with which patients find it challenging to cope. If sleep evades her due to being over-tired, she tries the simple pleasure of reading a book in order to relax and quiet her mind. She also takes an anti-fatigue pill at least once a day; more often than not she takes two. And when she gets more than eight hours of sleep, she feels excessively tired the follow day, proving it's a delicate balance to discover what works for your individual body.

She doesn't focus on nutrition, although she has made some small, sustainable choices in her diet that lead to lasting benefit. For example, she drinks lots of water, eats lots of vegetables and replaces at least one meal a day with a smoothie or shake. And although she drinks lots of coffee due to her very active lifestyle, by consuming lots of water she offsets it while staying properly hydrated. She selects foods that fuel her instead of making her feel sluggish, focusing on foods that minimize inflammation, admittedly not having found a specific diet that works for her, but just being informed about what she puts in her mouth because she is keenly aware that it will affect her in some way, physically speaking.

As far as being her own superhero and recognizing her resilience, her favorite quote by Uta Hagen says it all: "Overcome the notion that you must be regular. It robs you of the chance to be extraordinary."

***

Exercise is one of the more critical components in taking action toward being your own superhero and living well with chronic disease. The human body is designed to move, and although you may not do it perfectly or "right," something is better than nothing... everything in moderation... do the best you can. A strong body helps keep you well.

When you go to a public gym you will find many weight-training and/or exercise programs that are unfortunately one-size-fits-all. Most people, especially those over the age of 50, require a tailored, individualized program to focus on their personal goals. It's imperative to think about what goals *you* want to achieve and what intentions *you* want to set versus those indicated on a standardized chart. Have you ever considered what you want to do with your good health and strength? Fitness is very individualized, and finding a trainer to help get you started is one of the most beneficial ways to focus on your specific needs. Make a commitment to yourself to get in shape and be fit for you. And so that you don't slack off, work it into your schedule by making it an appointment on your calendar and finding a friend to be your exercise buddy and accountability partner.

Working with a trainer helps you stick to a routine because your trainer will create a program appropriate for you as well as provide the component of accountability. Besides, you'll likely keep an appointment, or at least think twice before canceling. When working with a trainer you won't overdue because they are monitoring you, so you won't fall off the bandwagon due to fatigue, soreness or overexertion. Start slowly, especially during the first month, taking baby steps to maintain enthusiasm without overdoing it. You want to avoid burnout and injury. Most people want a quick fix or a right-now result, but be realistic. It takes time to undo the damage you've done if you've been inactive for months or years. Professionals can help you set reachable and realistic goals, focus on a mind-body connection and validate that it's okay to take time to achieve success.

A trainer also provides various routines to always keep things interesting and switched up, combating muscle memory so you are always challenged. You seek out professionals for other types of health concerns, why not do so for exercise? As you age, life can become more difficult, and you have more physical limitations or issues that need accommodating. Now is always a good time to rethink how to be healthy for the rest of your life. It's okay to slow down when you feel it necessary; just don't stop!

There are varying opinions about what form of exercise is the most beneficial, but focus on something that you will actually do rather than just think about doing. (Consider how many people join a gym yet never go – certainly that's not helpful.) Performing a cardio workout to get to your *target heart rate* burns fat. Weight training builds muscle and strengthens bones. Most believe that a mix of the two is important. Your individual body dictates what combination works best for you. As an added bonus, start a regular practice of yoga, stretching, tai chi or another invigorating mind-body practice to help relieve stress, lengthen your muscles and increase your flexibility. All aid in lowering stress as well as play a role in preventing falls.

If you're thinking that your chronic disease prevents you from being able to exercise, consider this compelling story:

A woman started her career in the fashion industry, modeling, managing and working in boutiques; buying; coordinating fashion shows; etc. She was diagnosed with rheumatoid arthritis at the very young age of 20. At the time she didn't know what it meant and didn't care to find out. She found it extremely hard to accept that she was not perfect; although no one is, the fashion business is all about being perfect. Given this, she ignored it and hoped it would go away, but it didn't. Then she had to start seeing a rheumatologist. The doctor put her on medication, and friends who simply didn't understand thought it was horrible that she had to take medicine for the rest of her life. She actually thought it was fantastic that there was something to minimize her pain and help her feel better, although she was still in denial about having a chronic disease.

Eventually she recognized that she could no longer keep up with the fast-paced life of travel, work and needing to look perfect all the time. Extreme fatigue got in the way of her job and she couldn't go out and socialize as necessary, making her angrier and angrier. At the age of 40 she was forced to retire because she became quite ill, spending the majority of her day unable to get out of bed. Getting up or going out was a big deal and took vast amounts of effort. She was still smoking and her drink of choice was Diet Coke®.

A new doctor came into the picture and encouraged her to work with the arthritis foundation. She began to take classes, spent time in gyms and took note of how poor the personal training was. As she improved her personal health habits, she had the notion that she could work as a trainer to help people with health issues like hers, personalizing programs to fit their limitations. Working with a lot of different people with various medical issues gave her tremendous personal satisfaction. And as she discovered her superpower of resilience, she found it heartwarming to know she was making a difference helping others feel better and have a better quality of daily living.

Be aware that gyms are not always the answer. People respond differently to different atmospheres. For example, I cannot stand being in a gym. My senses are too vulnerable to the bright, harsh lights and loud sounds. I much prefer exercising outside in Mother Nature's gym. The important component is the trainer, wellness coach or exercise partner. That person acts as your accountability buddy, keeping you on track for achieving your fitness goals as well as teaching you how to do it properly so as to avoid injury.

I am often asked the question "If you're not feeling well, do you work out and push through it or do you take the day off?" The answer lies in the situation and in the individual person. If you tend to use not feeling well as an excuse, it is probably best to push yourself to work out. But if you really don't feel well or have a fever, it is probably best to rest. And if you think you might have an infection or a serious issue, call your doctor and do what they recommend. Don't beat yourself up if you miss a day or two. We are all human. Release your anger or disappointment in yourself and get back to it.

Sometimes fatigue is the obstacle. For those of you who are not familiar with clinical fatigue, it's not just about being tired; it's about being thoroughly unable to go one step farther because you have no more energy left in your tank. When you suffer from chronic disease, chances are that you face fatigue on a daily basis. I like to believe that I can do anything, just not everything. And like the story of the big rocks in the glass jar I told earlier, start with the important or necessary tasks so as to have enough energy to complete them, and possibly some leftover for other tasks. The important thing is to use your energy wisely so you always have enough to accomplish what's important to you.

It's imperative to get a release from your doctor before starting any exercise routine, even with a trainer. The American Council on Exercise recommends this, especially for people over the age of 40 and those in physical therapy. If you take beta blockers or have atrial fibrillation (a-fib), be aware that you cannot exercise at what is considered a normal target heart rate for your age; the medication and/or disorder prevent this, so it is vital to disclose what is going on with your health and any injuries you have to your doctor and trainer. Always share complete information; you know your body best.

If you want to work with a trainer, the best way to find one who fits your needs is to work with the person once or twice before purchasing an entire package of workouts. Make sure they keep your goals on the agenda and that you like them, so you look forward to doing the workout. Like trying a new hairdresser, it might take a few tries before finding the perfect trainer for you. Don't give up; you will find a good fit. Be sure they are certified by a reputable organization and ask for references. Look around the gym and see if people like you are working out. You want to feel comfortable where you're going without feeling competitive with anyone but yourself. Most people with chronic disease need a moderate cardio and weight-training program in order to avoid injury and/or fatigue. Avoid boredom by breaking up your routine into 10-minute segments by changing machines and inserting some brief stretching movements. Look forward to feeling better when you finish due to the release of endorphins (chemicals in your brain) that bring about feelings of euphoria, even if you start with an "I don't wanna do this" attitude. That will be your motivation to keep going back for more.

CHAPTER 13

SPIRITUALITY – ENERGY AND GRATITUDE

When one door closes another door opens,
but we so often look so long and so regretfully upon the
closed door that we do not see the ones which open for us.
– Alexander Graham Bell

She Not Only Survived Breast Cancer, She Thrived

A 50-year-old female Baby Boomer who was premenopausal discovered a lump in her breast and immediately sought care. After absorbing the shock of her diagnosis of cancer, she went into action, choosing to treat this horror as a challenge that she was going to beat. She made it her job to learn all that she could and to formulate an attack that would kill the beast without devastating her body more than necessary. She asked questions, read books, interviewed surgeons and oncologists and toured hospital treatment rooms. She first needed surgery, followed by weeks of chemotherapy and radiation: the best course of action to deter the cancer from metastasizing elsewhere in the future.

For the first years following her treatment she was very focused on nutrition, exercise and self-care. As time went by and she began to feel more like a normal person instead of a cancer patient, she cut back on her cancer-prevention practices, retreating to old, familiar habits that were easy and comforting. She kept up with her healthy eating because that made her feel physically better and she was losing the weight she had gained during chemotherapy. However, her exercise routine was still quite the challenge due to excessive fatigue, even though she no longer felt sick.

Throughout her treatment she was very cognizant of keeping her stress level to a minimum. She did this by reaching out to others who had had similar experiences in order to learn, get clear and increase her understanding of what to expect, the unknown becoming more familiar. Her brother and husband stepped in to take over her daily chores and responsibilities when needed to alleviate the self-inflicted stress of feeling that she was expected to do it all.

Another way she kept stress at bay was to try to be in control of what she could. She had specific friends for specific types of support she needed. For example, when she had her head shaved and went wig shopping, she included her fun, girly-stuff friends who would make the outing enjoyable without focusing on her being sick. She kept a separate list and schedule for those who took her to her treatments that provided her with a sense of increased security and decreased anxiety because she picked family and friends on whom she could rely without question. One time when I took her to a treatment, she cried and apologized for being emotional. Wanting to comfort her, I validated her feelings, told her she had nothing to apologize for, that this situation sucked, that she could lean on me for strength when needed and that together (along with her family and friends) we'd get her through this nightmare. You can't do this with everyone because you worry that it will hurt them too much if you show emotion, and you don't need any extra worry when you're physically and emotionally vulnerable. But you can do it with those you believe can handle it, who truly understand, who are empathetic to your plight. Find those family members and friends to help you and you'll get through anything.

A rare yet important action that helped her get through her experience with cancer was that she embraced being sick. Instead of seeing breast cancer as a negative from a victim point of view, she accepted it as how she was supposed to behave and gave herself permission to do what was necessary to feel well, like napping, relaxing and enjoying the small things in life. She released the need to do it all. Though she found it hard to focus on herself instead of others, over time she learned it was essential to do so. And with the support of empathetic friends, she was validated for doing that.

Her husband wanted to fix things, as many men do – it's in their emotional genetic programming. And even though he couldn't fix this, he always stayed positive – realistically, not like a Pollyanna – remaining practical, always having a positive perspective and taking care of things when needed without being asked until she was able return to her normal activities.

She opted not to have her husband take her to her chemo treatments because he was doing so much else. And as long as her friends were available to do so, she didn't want to burn him out. This way he was able to save his sick days and personal days off for more serious surgeries, procedures and setbacks. His going to work every day gave them both a sense of normalcy, which was important to their wellness.

After a few years she no longer thinks about cancer all the time. She has gone back to living her life, working full time and enjoying her time off with family and friends. What primarily helped her get through this crisis and come out stronger was her faith (or spirituality). She had always been a spiritual person with a strong sense of faith, though she was inconsistent in her practice of it. She always said her prayers at night to connect to God/Spirit/Energy, but after her treatments life got in the way and her spiritual practice slowly disappeared. Missing this important piece of herself, she has begun to take note of every day when she wakes up and to be very grateful for everything, from the most simple to the more complex. She's begun to regularly recite her prayers again at night before she goes to sleep, feeling more connected to God/Spirit/Energy once again. She and I regularly discuss healing prayer, its power and how to perform it daily, slowly adding it to her daily regimen so she can know she is healed physically and spiritually.

Along with her increased spirituality has come a strengthened attitude of gratitude. She has always been a generous person, and being faced with this challenge increased her desire to be grateful as well as to give back. She is a champion for those who need one, as well as for herself, always giving much and going that extra mile to help others in need. Perhaps if she had not experienced this unexpected turn of events, she might never have been awakened to this renewed sense of connectedness to community and spirit.

Spirituality: Tikkun Olam and Gratitude

Tikkun olam, literally meaning "repair of the world," is the Reform Judaism concept of living a meaningful life filled with giving and receiving, also known as social justice. It is based on the belief that by being grateful one can transform, repair and heal the world, and that by doing so one will also heal themselves.

As I mentioned earlier, in his book *When Bad Things Happen to Good People* Rabbi Harold Kushner discusses the randomness of the universe and the fact that no one and no great power controls what happens to you. Given such randomness, what matters most for a well-lived life is what you do with what happens to you: namely, your purpose (or what I like to call your destiny). Simply put, it's not what happens to you in life that matters; it's how you respond to it and how you use your unique gifts or superpowers to help others. This reminds me of the adage attributed to St. Ignatius: "Pray as if everything depends on God, act as if everything depends on you." The breast-cancer survivor did just that.

Tikkun olam teaches about finding your purpose, contributing to the greater good, having an attitude of gratitude, and how these qualities and attitudes impact your overall wellness. Life is hard, and this world can be a very difficult place to navigate. People can be mean and so stressed out that they live on autopilot until some crisis wakes them from their stupor. One small, simple action you can take today is to offer someone a compliment. You never know how much a few positive words can mean to someone. They might be going through something extremely difficult, and when you put your positivity out there in the universe, you might just neutralize that and make them happier. As a side effect, you become happier, too! Change someone's life with a random act of kindness; change your own. As Maya Angelou once said, "I've learned that people will forget what you said, people will forget what you did, but people will never forget how you made them feel." And honestly, you won't forget how you made them feel either; we are, after all, each a mirror to each other's souls.

A Paradigm for Spiritual Wellness

To create a paradigm for your spiritual wellness it is essential to live an inspired life, being the change you wish to see in the world. But that sometimes is easier said than done. To achieve this, begin by asking yourself, "Am I living my dreams now or putting them off until later? Am I inspired?" Becoming inspired is not a destination; it's a journey – much like the superhero journey. You are being called to something much deeper than your everyday life activities that you perform on autopilot, and to find that deeper meaning or purpose you must keep pursuing and risking while following what your heart really wants.

In his book *Inspiration Deficit Disorder*, Jonathan Ellerby discusses reconnecting to your inner sense of direction – a sense of knowing on a regular basis, slowing down and listening to that voice inside. He stresses trusting your gut and not allowing fear, negative expectations or your inner critic to stop you from forward momentum.

It's natural to strive for achieving perfection even though everyone falls short of that impossible goal. Although made with good intentions, perfection is not achievable; only your own personal excellence is. It is totally okay to strive for excellence rather than perfection – that's being human, which is actually super important! It's normal to experience bad days, pain and suffering, but when you are present and inspired you consider such negatives in the context of your choices and conscious decisions. A paradigm for wellness can include illness. For example, Gandhi might have suffered a stomachache from time to time, and the Dali Lama might get the flu. This is not about the end of pain or illness, but having a new relationship to them – a greater sense of peace, coherency and satisfaction.

As you live a busy life, striving for perfection, you tend to disconnect from yourself and your spirit, causing a lack of emotional connectedness. According to Ellerby, this emotional deficit is the breeding ground for lack of energy or lack of your life force. The congruency of your life – how your sense of passion, enjoyment and authenticity work together – is what manages your energy. The more you have of those, the more energy you have to address the challenges in your life. You may not realize it, but studies have shown that a vast number of visits to the doctor are due to stress-related conditions. Stress is the biggest contributor to personal suffering. And as I've said before, you have choice in regard to how much stress you allow into your life. If you eat a little differently, move a little more and take action to de-stress through a spiritual practice, you can save a lot of money on sick care.

Now is the time to put quality of life over quantity of life, redefining success not as the size of your paycheck or the number of hours you work, but as a life well lived. When you connect to what's important and experience lower stress and a higher level of satisfaction, you simplify your life, release frustration and find happiness within. You also discover your inner superpower of resilience. When faced with challenges, you learn and grow, taking a long look at what's in your heart and recognizing what's missing. Throughout life you are shaped by your disappointments, fears and obstacles. When you socialize with like-minded people and look inward via meditation, yoga, exercise and sleep, you reconnect to who you really are and what you really want.

Thousands of people regularly flock to speakers who talk about living inspired, and many invest hundreds of dollars in their programs in the hope of feeling connected to something greater than themselves. However, most people say that they already know how to feel inspired and connected. So why do they keep spending money to hear and learn? What might be holding you back from achieving inspiration and connection? The true barrier is you. Your gremlin might be causing you to think negatively. Become emotionally vigilant and open to understanding yourself on a deeper level. Part of you is wounded, filled with judgment and self-criticism (your gremlin). The other part of you is fundamentally wise, providing you with the confidence and resilience to be invincible. In the tradition of Buddhism, follow your wise self to move beyond suffering, and make choices rooted in doing the right thing. Although change is difficult, when you move toward it you are on the right track for positive growth and learning.

When you begin a spirituality practice, remember to keep it simple. Use deep breathing, appreciate silence and clear your mind. Take a step back from your life and learn to respond instead of react. Recognize that everything in life is based on energy. Good or positive energy raises you up; bad or negative energy drains you, leaving you sad and sick. Reconnect to yourself; replenish your soul.

Healing may not be so much about getting better,
as about letting go of everything that isn't you – all of the
expectations, all of the beliefs – and becoming who you are.
– Rachel Naomi Remen

Healing Touch

Healing touch is a form of energy healing. It is a holistic approach to healing that addresses who you are and what you're experiencing specific to you, your goals and your intentions. It offers pain relief; clearing and balancing of your chakras, or your energy; calms your nervous system; decreases anxiety; and opens you up spiritually and energetically. When performed, there is a partnership between client and practitioner that empowers the client to say, "This is what I need," and the practitioner to create an environment in which that particular healing can occur – to "open a space" for it. Healing is about balance. Healing touch addresses how trauma, no matter the size, impacts who you are and how it affects your energy. The human energy system includes:

- Meridians, which are pathways in the body along which vital energy is believed to flow. There are twelve such pathways in the human body, each associated with specific organs.
- Seven main chakras, each a vortex of energy that's like a three-dimensional spinning wheel of light that constantly contracts and expands, and each connected to a physiological function in the body

- An aura – your individual essence – which is generated by the movement of your chakras
- A universal energy field through which you can channel energy in a heart-centered way that regulates the flow of energy through your body (known in traditional Chinese healing as *chi*)

Your Seven Chakras

Chakras are the centers or locations in your body through which energy regularly flows. If one or more chakras are blocked, the lack of energy flow can lead to illness; hence it is beneficial to keep them "clear" so energy can flow freely throughout your body. Remember, everything is energy – even you.

1. **Root chakra:** where your sense of being grounded is centered, located at the base of your spine in your tailbone.

2. **Sacral chakra:** where your connection to others, or socialization, is centered, located just below your navel.

3. **Solar plexus chakra:** where your capacity to be confident and in control of your life is centered, located in your upper abdomen.

4. **Heart chakra:** where your ability to love and experience peace is centered, located just above your heart

5. **Throat chakra:** where your ability to express yourself authentically is centered, located in your throat.

6. **Third eye chakra:** where your ability to focus using intuition and wisdom, trusting your gut, is centered, located between your eyes.

7. **Crown chakra:** The highest chakra, representing your ability to be fully spiritually connected to the universe and its energy, is located at the crown or top of your head.

The universe is filled with energy, or *chi*. It is in and around everything, including you. As your vital life force, it enables you to think, breathe, move and live. Many people do not define energy as such because they cannot see it. But I have a sort of parlor trick that shows that a person has energy. I use a metal pendulum, or a necklace containing metal and/or a crystal. (You can even string together a bunch of paperclips.) You hold the pendulum loosely at one end as you emotionally release any desired outcome; there is a higher order of healing at play and you don't want to influence the pendulum with your own energy. Be sure to stay grounded, keeping your arm and hand still, while allowing the other end of the pendulum to hover over any one of someone's seven chakra points. Within a matter of seconds you will see the pendulum move. If it rotates in a clockwise circle it reveals an open chakra. If it is still or moves in a slow, vertical or counterclockwise direction, it shows the chakra is energetically compromised. If it moves at a good clip it shows a healthy, open and balanced chakra, representing free-flowing energy in that person's body.

Before you try this, I caution you that if you're doing it with someone whose energy is completely blocked, they might become hostile or angry when the pendulum doesn't move. When you first start trying this I suggest you choose only volunteers who seems open to the process or you might find yourself in an uncomfortable position.

To open the chakras energetically, healing touch releases the emotional anxiety tied to fear or worry. Prior to a healing-touch session, your practitioner discusses with you how you are feeling and helps you set an intention for the session. Being intentional, present and grateful enhances the practice and its efficacy. They then clear the air and clear your body of negative or blocked energy, slowly working through your body's energy system to heal and repair. In her article "How to Clear Your Chakras and Free Your Energy," on the Chopra Center's website, Tamara Lechner suggests other ways to get your energy flowing if your chakras are blocked. These tips include spending time in nature, especially walking barefoot so as to root down and connect with the earth. Other methods include eating foods and wearing clothes of the color associated with the particular blocked chakra; feeding or nourishing your body with what it tells you it's lacking; and spending time meditating, praying and/or chanting to activate your inner vibration, connect your chakras and get your energy flowing.

Energy healing is based on the supposition that
illness results from disturbances in the body's energies and
energy fields and can be addressed via interventions into
those energies and energy fields.
– Jed Diamond

When you practice gratitude, focus on your spirituality, experience healing touch, and/or energetically nourish your body with what it's missing, you promote healing because these all relax the body, stimulate healthy cell growth, release toxins, regulate the immune system and reconnect you to your inner life force, or *chi*. In a nutshell, they influence every cell in your body!

Your New Normal

Everybody likes an extraordinary person or likes to think that they would be great with a superpower in an ordinary world.
– Samuel L. Jackson

CHAPTER 14

SPIRITUALITY –
HEALING PRAYER

God/Energy is in everything and everything is in
God/Energy. God/Energy is the being that unites all of us.
We are all One. There is only God/Energy.
– Rabbi Douglas Goldhamer

A Rabbi's Journey through Healing Prayer

Many years ago, when modern medicine could not offer a sound resolution to his disease, a rabbi sought out healing prayer, known through Jewish mysticism and the prayer of the Kabballah. He suffered from a rare blood-clotting disease and was in extreme pain, and the doctors' medical solution was to amputate his legs in order to prevent death, but he didn't want to lose his legs due to the possibility of gangrene or infection. He heard of a Christian healer who might have a different solution, but asked him to refer him to a Jewish healer because as a rabbi he was uncomfortable with the notion of using Christian prayer to heal. He was referred to a well-known Hasidic healer who taught him healing prayer. This Hasidic healer showed him where it was written that healing is an art practiced by rabbis since the sixteenth century, and how valuable and important it is. Spiritual healing is a critical component to combine with modern medicine to create healing. Although he had used crutches to walk, after one year of praying (over 25 years ago) he was totally physically active without crutches and had no pain and no blood-clotting issues. This inspired him to pursue the study of spiritual healing more deeply and to become a healer to follow his *tikkun* of healing others.

Spirituality

How does spirituality play into taking action and becoming your own superhero? Among the dimensions of well-being is spirit. You have an awareness of a benevolent force that is greater than you that acts as the foundation of your mind-body-spirit connection. And through a spiritual belief or practice incorporated into your superhero journey, you can become a spiritual warrior who practices compassion, takes responsibility for your actions, is persistent and patient, speaks the truth, sets boundaries and does the hard or difficult thing when challenged. Spirituality is a major component of becoming your own superhero that comes to your rescue when times get tough. The bottom line is that it's all about love – loving others and loving yourself. And as an added bonus, spirituality also builds brain health!

Spirituality is not necessarily based in religion, but can be, depending on your beliefs. Think about a moment when you felt as if you were hanging on by a thread. I know that's how I felt when I first received my diagnosis; it felt like an insurmountable task just to get through the day. Some people turn to God through prayer for help. Others seek Spirit or simply look within for the energy to feel empowered to cope. Whatever your choice, it is right for you.

As a spiritual warrior you possess the divine qualities of kindness, empathy and doing the right thing regardless of fear; and you learn from your misfortunes. You might even say you are a conduit for the universe's positive energy, responding to life rather than reacting to it. Most important, when you strengthen your spirituality you learn to surrender to and trust the process called life. I am reminded of the "Serenity Prayer," first used in a sermon by the American theologian Reinhold Niebuhr: "God, grant me the serenity to accept the things I cannot change, courage to change the things I can, and wisdom to know the difference."

Ways you can strengthen your spirituality include:

- Developing a regular spiritual practice involving prayer, meditation or even yoga
- Listening to and trusting your heart, allowing yourself to feel your emotions and letting them guide you
- Always living in gratitude, recognizing that you are never alone

If you are still doubtful about whether or not you are (or can be) spiritual, consider this: A well-known twentieth-century philosopher, Rabbi Abraham Joshua Heschel, regularly began his lectures by stating, "A great miracle has just occurred." Audience members would gasp, their curiosity piqued. After a brief pause Rabbi Heschel would go on to say that the sun had just set. Everyone would shake their heads questioning how that was considered a miracle. Then he would speak about what he called "radical amazement": viewing the world in a way that takes nothing for granted and seeing God in everything. Everything is phenomenal; everything is incredible; always be in awe. To be spiritual is to be amazed. Even the simplest event like a sunset can be seen as incredible, worthy of amazement, if you are spiritual. So I challenge you to witness Mother Nature at work the next time you are outdoors or looking through a window, and tell me if you're not amazed. And when you are, I conclude you are also spiritual.

Healing Prayer

What is prayer? As found in Alice Calaprice's book *Dear Professor Einstein: Albert Einstein's Letters to and from Children,* in response to being asked if scientists pray, Albert Einstein replied:

Scientists believe that every occurrence, including the affairs of human beings, is due to the laws of nature. Therefore, a scientist cannot be inclined to believe that the course of events can be influenced by prayer, that is, by a supernaturally manifested wish. However, we must concede that our actual knowledge of these forces is imperfect, so that in the end the belief in the existence of a final, ultimate spirit rests on a kind of faith. Such belief remains widespread even with the current achievements in science. Everyone who is seriously involved in the pursuit of science becomes convinced that some spirit is manifest in the laws of the universe, one that is vastly superior to that of man.[18]

Einstein believed that prayer is based on our faith in something greater and has the power to uplift our spirit.

I learned of healing prayer through the rabbi mentioned at the beginning of this chapter. In 2003 my father received a diagnosis of thymic carcinoma, a very rare cancer of the thymus gland. Although my mother did not believe in healing prayer at the time, my father always claimed that he had a personal relationship with God and that they spoke often. This faith prompted my parents to pray with the rabbi prior to my father's surgery. Both of my parents prayed (and cried) in front of the ark with the rabbi. They claimed it was a spiritual experience like no other that reduced their stress while my father successfully underwent surgery and a lengthy recovery.

Until 2007 I had witnessed healing prayer from the sidelines. It worked for others, yet I wasn't really convinced. I actually was quite skeptical of all Judaism because my beliefs did not correlate to the prayers spoken in services on a regular basis. I was much more spiritual than religious, but had not come to that awareness – yet. Then in April of 2006, when MS entered my life, my perspective began to shift. After taking almost a full year to adjust physically to the medication and my new lifestyle, I called the rabbi. He welcomed me with open arms, immediate unconditional love and a non-obtrusive sensitivity that no one else had ever shown me aside from my parents.

Our first visit was awkward, as I did not know what to expect. When he asked about my expectations, my explanation was that it would work like therapy; he would listen to me and use rabbinical thought and traditions to explain why I felt the way I did. He promptly told me with a glint in his eye, "No, it doesn't work that way. This is not therapy. I am not a shrink." We shared a laugh and then I hesitantly asked, "Then what exactly *is* healing prayer?"

We began discussing the power of healing prayer in others. He shared in-depth stories of people's tumors disappearing. Apparently people come from all over the world to pray with and learn from this rabbi because healing prayer works best when done regularly and with someone who is skilled. It is nowhere near as powerful when practiced alone. When participating in healing prayer it's important to also follow your physician's medical advice. Prayer does not replace prescribed medications or protocol. It is an addition to them.

Clarifying my beliefs was the next step. I was not sure I believed in God, specifically, but I did believe in a universal power greater than mankind. I define God as energy – a universal life force – versus a traditional human-like figure sitting on a throne up in heaven. Energy is not necessarily visible to the naked eye; however, everything is made up of energy. Fortunately for me, healing prayer is based on having faith in the energy of God. God is conscious-thinking, compassionate, giving energy. Humans are created in God's image, and God is present within all of us (and outside all of us). God is everywhere. Her energy is harnessed and activated through healing prayer.

There was a revealing experiment done by the University of Arizona in conjunction with the Global Consciousness Project regarding advances of consciousness and health. They examined correlations that reflected universal energy in the expression of global love, focusing on the date April 29th, 2011. That was the day Prince William and Kate got married. The energetic expression of global love was that of their kiss. They used a special device based in Arizona that tracked random activity of energetic electrons in the world. When William and Kate stepped out onto the balcony, energy levels increased. When the remainder of the royal family stepped out onto the balcony, energy levels increased even further. While they were standing there energy levels stayed relatively steady until there was a slight uptick, and that was when the crowd started chanting, "Kiss, kiss, kiss." When William and Kate demurely kissed, the crowd went wild, as shown through the energy indicator. Then the levels dropped a bit, staying steady. However, several minutes later researchers noticed a dramatic uptick. And what do you think this correlated to? The second kiss. For those of you who watched on TV, you know this second kiss was definitely more romantic than the first, and the crowd exploded with elation. Isn't it truly amazing that the energy levels of this crowd's consciousness in London were measured thousands of miles away in Arizona? Energy is universal; it is everywhere and in everything.

The pendulum trick I described earlier shows this as well. You might recall that if a person's energy is blocked the pendulum might not move, and you might wonder what causes a person to have low or blocked energy. The person might be sick or they might be keeping their emotions bottled up inside them. There are practitioners who do things like reiki, healing touch and various other forms of energy healing to clear blockages, primarily in the chakra points.

I believe that through meditation and/or prayer, energy can be harnessed to heal the mind and body. Many ancient cultures practice energy rituals such as chi gong, tai chi, yoga, meditation, healing prayer, etc. that have become popular in contemporary life due to their proven, positive, healing effects. When you practice any of these energy rituals, you allow your subconscious mind the ability to invite change so as to gain a greater sense of self and well-being.

Most problems and negative energy stem from your thinking. What you think affects how you feel, and how you feel affects how you behave. A regular spiritual practice helps you align with your inner core energy, shifting it to a higher level. It helps calm your mind, quiets inner thoughts, reduces stress and allows your truth to unveil itself as you focus inward. A regular spiritual practice helps connect the body and mind for optimal wellness.

To *meditate* literally means to think, contemplate, devise or ponder. It's a mental practice used for the purpose of experiencing heightened awareness within silence and relaxation, very similar to the heightened awareness of healing prayer. Scientists and physicians are researching the effects of meditation on the brain. Through MRI studies it has been proved that meditation positively affects the health of the brain. Studies are showing that a regular practice of meditation also:

- Promotes deep breathing, which stimulates blood flow and sends healing to your entire body
- Aids digestion
- Increases energy
- Reduces stress
- Reduces frequency of illness
- Improves memory
- Improves overall wellness

There are many types of meditation, but the true essence is the same: it involves intention, focus and deliberate breathing. Healing prayer also includes specific invocations to recite that help activate the cells within the body. It requires practice and dedication. Change does not happen overnight.

As I mentioned, I have practiced healing prayer regularly for over 10 years. Recently I combined this practice with yoga. I use the technique as a form of meditation that directs my thoughts inward energetically, helping me align my energy with that of the universe and God/Spirit/Energy.

Healing prayer is guided by the notion that one does not pray to be given strength; one prays to be healed. It uses principles embraced by the Christian and Jewish traditions for guiding our healing. Both faiths maintain that when you pray, you pray as if your prayer has already been answered. If you and God are focused on healing, you will be healed. Trust in your resilience and energy.

Practicing Healing Prayer

Healing prayer is based in biblical teachings and can be performed by anyone no matter their faith or religious belief. The only essential components are to believe in a power greater than you that is of both the feminine and masculine divine and that is in everything and every moment. When the feminine and masculine are metaphorically split, there is illness and disease, typically rooted in hate or negative energy. When united, there is healing and wellness, rooted in love or positive energy. And the key to uniting them is vibration.

When the world first began in the Garden of Eden, all was one. Then appeared a tree that was different: the tree of knowledge.

Once it was tasted, a separation between light and dark, sickness and wellness occurred and humans were exiled from the heavenly garden to the earthly world. The female divine left the male divine and went into every person's soul, while the male divine remained outside of the soul. This is why it is believed that we are all born with the feminine divine within us while the masculine divine transcends us. When the two divine presences are united within a person's soul, their energies come together, strengthening, transforming and healing. And remember, your body is made up of cells. Every cell has a soul that forms your entire soul.

The Hebrew word representative of the two aspects of God, or the Divine, is *Anochi* [ah-no-hee], a derivative of the word representing both the feminine and masculine. In order to perform healing prayer, you must imagine the feminine and masculine uniting, connecting you to your cells and your body.

Each of us is connected spiritually and energetically to the Divine in some fashion, and you become unified with it through your breath. Through breathing and focusing your thoughts in a specific manner, you activate your cells to vibrate energetically, thereby activating the presence of the Divine within you for healing.

I equate my interpretation of the Jewish technique of healing prayer to that of using your chakra points and your breath. Regardless of method, the goal is to activate your cells to vibrate in unison to stimulate healing in your body. When you are ill, your cells may not be vibrating strongly, much less in harmony. Healing takes place when the energy within you and outside of you (or the feminine and masculine divine) is actively pulsating in synchronization.

Now you are ready to practice healing prayer. Again I caution you that healing prayer is to be performed in conjunction with advice from your medical professional, not instead of it.

Start by loving and appreciating your body. Don't be mad at it for betraying you with sickness. Love it. Thank it. Recognize that each part of your body has a soul, even on the cellular level. Each organ and cell has a soul. These souls all desire love and compassion that you give them through positive self-talk, meditation and healing prayer. As you fill your mind, body and soul with positive energy, healing begins as the cells start to repair themselves. Pray with faith that your prayers have already been answered. Do so with gratitude and knowledge that every soul of every cell in your body is balanced, therefore healed.

Sit comfortably in a chair with your back straight and feet flat on the floor. Close your eyes and gently breathe, focusing on inhaling and exhaling through your nose. As you develop a rhythm, begin chanting either "Anochi" or "Om," slowly and specifically, enunciating each syllable. To enhance the strength of your energetic activation, if you're comfortable doing so you can say, "I place divine energy before me always," while feeling the vibration in each area of your body on which you are focusing, with a growing sense of pressure. Continue to do this while trying to actually see the light of the Divine in your mind's eye and feel its vibration. When your body is filled with light and all your cells are vibrating in unison, healing takes place. You and the Divine have become one. "I AM" is the phrase to think of, which acknowledges that you and the Divine are one. In the Hebrew Bible, "I AM" equates to the name of God and to your saying what you will do. The name for you and God is interchangeably I AM.

Healing Prayer through the Activation of Anochi

As previously mentioned, *Anochi* represents the activation of the feminine and masculine divine through Jewish healing prayer. You do not have to be Jewish to practice this form, but if you're not comfortable with it a Zen version using the activation of Om follows.

Dress in loose clothing that does not restrict breathing deeply. Sit comfortably with your back straight. Close your eyes. Focus on your breath. Be aware as you inhale and exhale.

Start with visualizing the crown or top of your head. Imagine a light entering and filling your body. Inhale, and as you exhale say, "I place God/Spirit/Energy before me always," while continuing to breathe. Repeat this for each of the following areas of your body:

Throat
Right shoulder
Left shoulder
Right arm
Left arm
Center of your chest at heart level
Upper abdomen or solar plexus
Lower abdomen or sacra
Tailbone
Right hip
Left hip

Now visualize the feminine and masculine divine together in each of your cells. To activate their vibrations, or energies, so they will be in unison to promote healing, focus on the word *Anochi*, representing both the feminine and masculine God/Spirit/Energy.

Be sure you are still sitting comfortably with your back straight, eyes closed. Breathe slowly and deeply, through your nose, in long breaths.

Now inhale through your nose, hold for a moment, and exhale through your mouth, making an "ah" sound, feeling its vibration in your mouth and deep inside your core.

Inhale through your nose again, hold for a moment, and on your next exhalation make a "noh" sound, feeling its vibration in your mouth and deep inside your core.

Inhale through your nose again, hold for a moment, and on your next exhalation make a "hee" sound, feeling its vibration in your mouth and deep inside your core.

Do this version of healing prayer 10 times, slowly and deeply.

You have filled yourself with God/Spirit/Energy's breath and healing energy, and both the feminine and masculine divine are now united, awakened and activated within you.

Once you have activated or awakened the Divine within you, if you wish to make your prayer even stronger, go through each section of your body again, saying aloud, "I send love, care and compassion to every cell of my [body

189

area]. I love the souls of the cells of my [body area]." This will inspire each soul of each cell to love, care, repair and heal itself.

If the Jewish form of healing prayer isn't congruent with your beliefs, when you focus your thoughts during meditation, yoga or any other spiritual practice, also focus on your breath, and when you exhale say aloud the Hindu word *Om* [ah-oh-um] as a sacred sound or mantra that unites the universe with your soul. *Om* also creates a vibration within to activate your energy on a cellular level.

Activating Your Energy through the Vibration of Om

Sit comfortably with your back straight. Close your eyes. Focus on your breath. Be aware as you inhale and exhale. Breathe slowly and deeply, through your nose, in long breaths.

Now inhale through your nose, hold for a moment, and exhale through your mouth, making an "ah" sound, feeling its vibration in your mouth and deep inside your core.

Inhale through your nose again, hold for a moment, and on your next exhalation make an "oh" sound, feeling its vibration in your mouth and deep inside your core.

Inhale through your nose again, hold for a moment, and on your next exhalation make an "um" sound, feeling its vibration in your mouth and deep inside your core.

Do this meditation 10 times; slowly and deeply.

You have filled yourself with God/Spirit/Energy's breath and you are now connected with the universe and its healing energy.

> *Energy flows where attention goes.*
> *– Michael Beckwith*

Healing prayer is based on the notion that life (or living) is your school. Although you are never separate from God/Spirit/Energy, you face hardships and struggles in order to learn how to heal not only yourself but others, too. Prayer and meditation make your growth possible, allowing for a vision or belief greater than you that nourishes your soul.

To gain the most benefit from healing prayer, practice it every day. Think of your spirituality (like your resilience) as a muscle that needs constant use to stay strong. Meditating and praying are like going to the spiritual gym – balancing your cells, protecting yourself from aging and illness and strengthening your ability to function from a source of love. Consider God/Spirit/Energy's presence in your life as a mirror: How it acts toward you is how you act toward others. Like the concept of karma – cause and effect, think of it as your magic elixir that you return with from your superhero journey to share with others. Instead of shutting down in the face of illness or aging, connect to the universe through vibration and breath. Heal yourself, heal God/Spirit/Energy within you and outside of you, and heal others. Become your own resilient spiritual warrior; be your own superhero.

Many texts teach how to heal through prayer and meditation rooted in the power of God/Spirit/Energy as a loving, compassionate energy open to all faiths. But the origin of healing prayer is different in different religions. There is no one perspective that is better than another. I focus on the Jewish version of healing prayer because it's familiar. The Jewish perspective is based on the Hebrew Bible, Book of Numbers, Chapter 12. In it Moses was chastised by his sister, Miriam, for marrying a woman who was black and not Jewish. Miriam and their brother, Aaron, were furious at the leader of the Hebrews for doing so. They gossiped about him, criticized him and chastised him, and it happened that Miriam, the leader of the movement against Moses, noticed her skin turning white as snow. It was as if God was saying, "You really like white, become white."

And she became white as snow, a symptom of leprosy in those days. Like cancer in modern times, leprosy was a horrific, incurable disease that many people were plagued with. It resulted from gossip, according to ancient rabbis.

Miriam told Moses she was plagued with this horrible leprosy, and he lifted his hand to God and said, "*El nah refa nah lah: Oh God, heal her now.*" He said these few simple words with force and belief, then took her to the priest/physician, who gave her medicine. Through medicine and prayer, Miriam was healed.

El nah refa nah lah became the basis for healing prayer in Judaism. Even though prayer is essential, it must be used in conjunction with a physician's assistance to result in miracles of healing, as it did with Miriam. She became completely healed, became a great prophet among the people of Israel, recognized her wrongdoing and became a role model.

Isaac Luria, a Jewish mystic considered the father of Kabbalah, wrote about praying as if your prayer has already been answered, and about the importance of being a giving and good person to strengthen the effectiveness of your prayer. When you help others, you also help and heal yourself. Pray in joy, not sadness, to show your faith, knowing you will be healed. Prayer is not reading from a book; prayer is an art with rules, and there are ways to perfect it. The more you study the rules of prayer and practice it, the better your practice will be. Remember, prayer is rooted in compassion, passion, visualization and faith.

All prayer is for healing; however, a cure is not always possible. You can live well with disease, which is healing. To be cured means you don't have to address your disease any longer. To be healed means you maintain a healthy life, keeping disease at bay while being nonsymptomatic and preventing disease from attacking your body again. Even with a disease that can be "cured" there is no guarantee that it won't come back. Being healed means that symptoms are not present.

How do you begin a practice of healing prayer, especially if you do not have a skilled clergyperson to whom to reach out? Although it is more efficacious if you seek out a practitioner, you can learn from a book (see "Suggested Resources" at the end of this book). First do what your physician tells you in regard to medication and/or therapy. Then pray. Use faith, happiness, visualization or any type of prayer, and you will be amazed by the results. Faith is a very important component of healing.

I believe in a universal principal that every person is created in the image of God/Spirit/Energy and is like God/Spirit/Energy. There is no separation between man and God/Spirit/

Energy. God/Spirit/Energy lives in each of us and in the plants, the sky, the earth, etc. We are all ONE regardless of religion. The entire universe is connected through the Divine. Although this divine principle is used in mystical Judaism, it is also embraced in Christianity. Jesus taught it.

When faced with adversity, recognize with confidence and faith that you have the ability to activate this divine principle within you, and be confident that you will be healed. Similar to electricity, the universe's energy lives in each individual. And as a light switch turns on a light, you turn on or activate the divine spirit within you. When you do, you have the power to overcome anything. We all struggle to know, and without knowing the answer we all strive to overcome obstacles. When you embrace this greater universal energy, you are able to conquer adversity.

You might be wondering about the difference between prayer and meditation. When praying, you are asking God/Spirit/Energy for something by activating the souls of your body's cells. When meditating, you are experiencing the presence of God/Spirit/Energy within you. Healing prayer and meditation, together, activate your divine energy, just as what you say after "I AM" does, shaping your reality, becoming indicative of your destiny.

CHAPTER 15

———

Putting Together
Your Superhero Team

When "I" is replaced by "we,"
even "illness" becomes "wellness."
– Malcolm X

In the past several chapters you have learned about an integrative approach to being proactive in your health care from various perspectives. Being mindful that no superhero ever works completely alone, always having at least one partner, friend or sidekick to assist and act as backup, now is the time to put together your own superhero team. This team will offer you expert assistance, guidance and nonjudgmental accountability while championing you to personal success. Using the structure of my team as an example, I hope you will find inspiration. Your team does not have to have all the members that mine does, and it can have more or different ones. Customize it to your needs. After all, it's YOUR team!

Superhero Team Members

The Gatekeeper: This ought to be your primary caregiver or internist. Together, you manage your overall health. They must listen to you, consulting other physicians in your team when necessary; keep you in check; and not allow you to dwell in bouts of denial, sadness or confusion especially to the point of causing undo stress. Choose a doctor who allows you to guide the conversation and tries to help you as best they can. Make sure they are trustworthy and be open and honest with them at all times. In today's health-care climate you really have to be your own advocate and speak up when you feel you need something, without exaggeration or hypochondria. You are the co-captain with your doctor. Remember that doctors are not gods, and medicine is still a *practice*. We're called patients to have patience with them and ourselves.

The Specialist: Your condition dictates what type of specialist you might require. MS is a neurologic autoimmune disease, so a neurologist is essential for me. A neurologist treats disorders that affect the brain, spinal cord and nerves: the central nervous system. My neurologist has been treating patients with MS for over 40 years and is expert in all things MS-related, medically speaking. If you have or had cancer, you would seek out an oncologist; heart disease, a cardiologist; etc. Choose someone who is open-minded to other approaches beyond the pharmacological and who supports your adherence to a disease-modifying therapy (medication) in addition to any mind-body-spirit, integrative lifestyle modifications you develop.

The Integrative Medicine Professional: This is a specialist who looks at you, your body and your health as a whole, using a combination of traditional and alternative medicine to help you achieve optimal health and healing tailored to you as an individual. Working with an integrative physician, you learn the importance of knowing your "numbers," including your blood values (such as vitamin-D level; C-reactive protein level, which measures inflammation; cholesterol level; etc.), blood pressure, pulse and weight, as well as how to integrate nutrition, exercise and spirituality as a healthy lifestyle. An integrative approach reveals an entirely new perspective for you that emphasizes the importance of proactive health care versus reactionary sick care. To find an integrative medicine professional in your area, search the University of Arizona Center for Integrative Medicine website at https://integrativemedicine.arizona.edu/alumni.html. If you cannot find an integrative practitioner where you live or it is too expensive to add one to your team, ask other team members if they can approach your care using a holistic or integrative modality.

The Nutritionist: This team member helps you learn about feeding your hunger for health, happiness and living life to the fullest. Remember, nutrition is not just about *what* you eat; it's also about *why* you eat. Brain receptors react to sugar and other "comfort" foods, fooling you about these foods making you feel better when in fact they only cause you to feel worse. Food also contributes to increased or decreased inflammation, and inflammation is the root of all disease. Consider your eating habits: whether you eat out of hunger or stress and what types of food choices you make based on convenience. Determine what foods you absolutely will and will not give up or modify so your nutritionist can create an eating plan that actually works for you, not against you. For example, I was not willing to give up coffee, wine or the occasional piece of dark chocolate. And that was okay. I learned that moderation was the key.

A nutritionist (or registered dietician) can teach you characteristics of an anti-inflammatory way of eating (important for someone with MS or other chronic disease) as well as clarify what foods are truly healthy, deciphering the realities behind advertisements and others' opinions. Using your blood's C-reactive protein level (C-RP) as the indicator of inflammation in your body, you can inquire about taking certain vitamins or supplements to help reduce inflammation if eating an anti-inflammatory diet is insufficient. These include turmeric, green tea extract, magnesium, vitamin B complex, a probiotic, and fish oil, to name a few. You might also add a daily serving of mixed berries to get plenty of antioxidants, which are important in offsetting the normal oxidative stress or deterioration of your body's cells, which happens quicker in less healthy bodies. If you take a large quantity of vitamins, ask how to incorporate them into your morning smoothie, creating a quick, easy and delicious anti-inflammatory cocktail.

The Exercise Physiologist: When faced with chronic disease, exercise can be daunting. It is all too common for people to purchase expensive gym memberships or equipment that go unused, wasting money and contributing to their ill health. And, unfortunately, there are many "trainers" out there who are not adequately certified to customize a workout to meet your special needs. It is imperative to do your homework and seek out a properly credentialed trainer such as an exercise physiologist. According to the American College of Sports

Medicine, "Certified Clinical Exercise Physiologists® (CEP) provide exercise-related consulting, and conduct assessments and individualized training to guide and strengthen the lifestyles of those with cardiovascular, pulmonary, and metabolic diseases and disorders."[19] Their training is exceptional and applicable to all sorts of people with chronic disease.

For example, many people with MS experience a temporary worsening of their symptoms when they overheat, whether due to weather, activity or experiencing a fever. Vision can become blurred, extremities can tingle, balance can be compromised and energy can decrease. Generally, heat usually produces only a temporary worsening of symptoms. Once temperature is regulated those symptoms dissipate. Figuring out how to exercise without overheating was challenging for me. Since my college days I adhered to the motto "No pain, no gain," and worked out with intensity. An exercise physiologist taught me how to do cardio in the form of *interval training* (revving up and cooling down) as well as to keep a fan on me when doing cardio or weight training so as not to overheat my body. He also taught me the importance of changing up routines to avoid boredom and my body getting accustomed to them so that I would continue to challenge my body and brain every time.

In order to not only maintain your strength and stamina with a chronic illness but also lower your C-RP and blood pressure while improving your heart and brain health, it is recommended to exercise at least 30 minutes, five or six times a week. Of course you might not be able to do this right away. And you may have to push yourself, which is okay as long as you are under the supervision of a professional to help guard against injury or worsening of symptoms. Set aside time for a nap to regain your energy to get through the day if you find exercise physically draining, as I often do.

The Energy Healer: Whether you choose yoga, meditation, reiki, healing touch, healing prayer or another energy-based modality, energy healing is an essential component of wellness. As previously discussed, you are energy; your cells are energy. When you are ill or stressed, your energy can be blocked or stagnant. By activating your energy you get it moving, causing cells to vibrate, thereby creating blood flow, which promotes healing.

I sought out a rabbi who is an expert in healing prayer, in addition to beginning a yoga practice, learning meditation and experimenting with healing touch. Although skeptical at first, I came to realize that all of these modalities, each in their own unique way, activate the cells in my brain and body to aid healing. They have also helped me strengthen my sense of faith in God/Spirit/Energy and in myself, playing a major role in my spiritual superhero journey to self-discovery.

The Rest of the Team: The rest of your team can include other practitioners such as a dentist, ophthalmologist, gynecologist, urologist, audiologist or dermatologist, as well as friends and family. Consider including creative art teachers, book group leaders and others who can teach you new activities to not only challenge your brain but nurture your natural desire for socializing and creativity. It truly takes a team to ensure you are well. You cannot nor should you have to do it alone. Choose your team members wisely, making sure they are properly credentialed and in line with your goals. Getting through life with chronic disease is challenging. With a knowledgeable team behind you offering tools, support, empathy and love, you can nurture and optimize your resilience throughout your journey.

The MOST Important Member: YOU! Your team starts and ends with you. You are in charge. You know what is best for you and how you truly feel. You know what motivates you and you are the only one who can choose to live well. You are your own superhero!

CHAPTER 16

═══

JUST FOR MEN

*Courage is not having the strength to go on; it is going on
when you don't have the strength.*
– Theodore Roosevelt

I include this special brief chapter for men because society
holds you up to a different standard than women. I recognize
that not all of the messages in this book resonate with you
because of this. With the ever-popular book by Dr. John Gray,
Men Are from Mars; Women Are from Venus, in mind, I'm sure
you often hear that women are emotional and men are not.
As a man you probably have been taught to be strong and
not show emotion, which is considered a sign of weakness.
And I doubt you cry to release emotions; or if you do, you
are uncomfortable doing so because crying is thought to
be taboo for men. A man symbolizes strength; king of his
castle, protector against all evil; a macho superhero. There
is no room for frailty of any sort, especially when you suffer
illness.

Okay, now that those stereotypes are out of the way, let's get real. You are a human being who experiences emotions just as anyone else, regardless of gender. Your mind, body and spirit need nurturing and care just as a woman's. And being proactive in regard to your health care provides a more positive outcome just as it does for women. But guess what? According to research published in the *Journal of Neurology* last year, men take longer than women to report symptoms and to get evaluated when ill. And this particular article specified that this was the case for men with symptoms of MS. It also said that men tended to start treatment later and had lower rates of adherence to disease-modifying therapies.

According to a NewsUSA online survey of current trends in men's health, one of the biggest obstacles to improving men's health care was men themselves. Among the findings was that 29 percent of men said they waited as long as possible before seeing a doctor when they felt sick, were in pain or were concerned about their health. It was also found that most men led sedentary lives with only 38 percent exercising on a regular basis.[20] The Centers for Disease Control and Prevention – National Center for Health Statistics estimated in a 2013-2014 study that more than 73 percent of men were overweight or obese.[21] These statistics are not good. So do I have your attention? Do you want to discover your superpower of resilience, too?

Just as I discussed throughout this book, you have all the power you need to be resilient using the tools presented as steppingstones. As an old American proverb states, the only difference between stumbling blocks and steppingstones is the way you use them. It is understandable that talking about your feelings or your issues of ill health is uncomfortable because you were taught not to do it. My suggestion is to seek out a male doctor and include close male friends on your team. Join a men's support group as an outlet for the negative emotions you are sorting through and a safe place to open up, where you can benefit from guy-talk and enjoy being part of a community away from the eyes of judgmental women (if there are any of those in your life). The term *male bonding* came to be for a reason. In a man-to-man friendship there is a bond that allows for straightforward conversation, nonjudgment and loyalty.

When you do finally open up about your disease you will most likely find you are filled with unresolved anger and frustration from your new limitations. Seek help from someone so you can learn how to release your anger and shift your thinking to the positive. When you normalize seeking out help from others, you become more accepting and forgiving of yourself, recognizing that you are, in fact, your own superhero without all the machismo – cape optional.

CHAPTER 17

―――――――――

ADVOCACY, PATIENT ADHERENCE AND SELF-CARE

Being a caretaker is [not], and never will be, an easy job;
in fact, it is that hardest job in the world and many times a
thankless job. You have to be the pillar of strength even when
you feel like you are crumbling to pieces inside.
— Jenna Morasca

Days run into nights filled with injections, blood draws,
catheter in/out/in, not eating/eating, walking/not walking,
bed/chair, sleeping some or not at all. After day six he finally
turns the corner after sleeping for almost 20 hours and his
kidneys are slowly starting to work properly. And after
quietly sneaking into his room at 5:30am, I hear the words
that reinforce my looking after him as the right thing to do:
"Your presence brings me comfort," he says as he briefly opens
his sleepy eyes and glances in my direction. Later, as I was
holding his stuffed heart pillow, I said, "I'm holding your
heart, you know." And he replied, "You do," with a smile and

a familiar twinkle in his eye. At that moment my exhaustion melted away without another thought.

Regardless of whether or not you have close relationships with family and friends, when you are going through a trauma you need to either advocate for yourself or have someone do it for you. As the woman who survived breast cancer said, "I think cancer is a hard battle to fight alone or with another person at your side, but having someone to pick you up when you fall and stand by your side through every appointment and delivery of bad news is priceless." It is invaluable to have another person listen to what your doctor says and ask questions you might not think of. It is imperative to be the "squeaky wheel," advocating for yourself when things don't progress or get done in accordance with your expectations. And it is always priceless to have someone help pick up the pieces should you fall apart when hearing devastating and/or unexpected news.

Advocacy

When in the hospital or going to a doctor's appointment, it is always beneficial to take someone with you. For example, when I went to an appointment with a specialist for a second opinion prior to my definitive diagnosis, I knew I would shut down if I heard bad news. I knew I needed someone there with me. So I took reinforcements with me in the form of my family. They listened intently when I could not. They asked questions that I did not consider. They kept open a space in the room for me to have my meltdown and rejoin the conversation when I was ready. They prevented the doctor from assuming we were finished and leaving before we understood everything we needed to and what the next steps were.

When choosing those who will champion on your behalf, consider that they:

- Know your wishes and needs and won't confuse them with their own. If they don't know, they need to ask you or you need to tell them. Write it down if necessary.
- Will ask questions and keep clarifying until they and you understand absolutely everything. There are no trivial or dumb questions.
- Will keep track of all pertinent information including test results, medications, treatment options, treatment decisions and appointment dates in an organized manner.
- Are trustworthy, have good communication skills and are super dependable. Trust them with your life. Consider them to be your superhero when you are unable to be your own.

Have a privacy authorization form and/or medical power of attorney drawn up under Health Insurance Portability and Accountability Act (HIPAA) parameters for each person you take with you to your appointments. The Health Insurance Portability and Accountability Act of 1996 provides data privacy and security provisions for safeguarding medical information. Such authorization allows them to participate in all medical conversations and make necessary decisions in the event you are incapacitated.

As human beings we value the experience that comes with age. We are reminded over and over again that our elders should be cherished and respected by sayings like "older and wiser" and "respect your elders." Whether you are a Millennial or Gen Xer focused on building your career, or an aging Baby Boomer planning for your golden years, you might not appreciate the value of having respect for your elders because life is going by at an alarming rate of speed. But when you become impaired by chronic disease, everything slows down or even comes to an abrupt halt. Sadly, though, your memory and ability to respond also slow down as you age; it happens to the best of us. But consider what I said before – every superhero has a backup: Superman had Lois, Batman had Robin, and the list goes on. Going it alone is not a sign of strength, and asking for help is not a sign of weakness. You are human, and it's perfectly normal to be completely freaked out during a crisis. Having a close confidant to support you makes all the difference in the world, in a good way.

Self-Advocacy

Advocating for yourself is something most people are afraid to do because it seems outside the box of being nice and polite as forceful or too brazen. But being subtle or restrained sometimes doesn't get results. I'm not saying you have to be mean or hostile; you have to be persistent and not give up in the face of unresponsiveness. I waited by the phone for two months to hear from the pharmaceutical company that was arranging testing and first-dose observation for a new medication my doctor prescribed. Every week I emailed the doctor's nurse stating I had not heard anything. Distressed, I found a phone number and called them myself. It turned out that my case was considered closed and no one was working on anything! Immediately I emailed my doctor's nurse and she agreed that was unacceptable and promised to pursue getting the situation rectified. Imagine what might have happened had I not made that call. Most likely no one would have reached out to me, I would have given up and remained on my current medication, and my doctor would have been completely unaware of the situation until my next checkup. Worst of all, I could have experienced a flare-up because my current medication was not working as well as it should have. If I had not advocated for myself, I might have gotten sicker.

In today's hectic world you have but few precious moments when visiting your doctor. So it's imperative to arrive prepared and not waste valuable time. As part of your self-advocacy, here are a few best practices to consider:

- Prepare a list of questions in writing so you can write down the answers next to the questions.
- Prepare a list of current medications, including vitamins and supplements, and their corresponding dosages.
- Share your health history, including allergies, illnesses and surgeries.
- Take any x-rays, scans and test results your physician might not have.
- Wear your glasses and/or hearing aids, if needed.
- Dress appropriately and be clean and neat, showing you care.
- Arrive early with insurance card in hand to fill out necessary paperwork.
- Be truthful and thorough.

- Take a trusted family member or friend if you are nervous or feel you won't pay close attention to what is being said.
- If you're afraid to talk to your doctor, consider getting a new one. This is one of the most trusted relationships you should have!

Patient Adherence

Patient adherence also plays a vital role in your health care. The World Health Organization found:

> Among patients with chronic illness, approximately 50% do not take medications as prescribed. This poor adherence to medication leads to increased morbidity and death and is estimated to incur costs of approximately $100 billion per year. Today's ever more complicated medical regimens make it even less likely that physicians will be able to compel compliance and more important that they partner with patients in doing what is right together.[22]

Your physician is the "gatekeeper" on your team and YOU are the co-captain. You need to work together to maintain adherence to your disease-modifying therapy in addition to other beneficial integrative practices to produce the best possible outcome.

If remembering to take your medications is a problem, here are a few suggestions to help trigger your memory:

- Use an inexpensive pill organizer. They come in a variety of styles to help you organize your medications by day and time.

- Place your medications where you will see them. When they are no longer in sight, you'll know you've taken them.
- Try a reminder app on your cell phone that provides a ringtone to alert you to the time to take your medicine.

People often tell me about mistakes hospitals make and how horrible they are, or how their doctor never called them back or read their chart, and all they do in response is sit around waiting for someone to contact them or make the situation better. You have to take control of your own care, or have someone you trust do it for you. You have to keep track of and question everything. Keep copious notes and copies of all test results. Be honest and straightforward. You were given two ears to listen and one mouth to talk, so listen more and talk less. When you see how fragile and delicate life can be, all the trivial chatter fades into the background while you focus on what truly matters: your wellness.

Self-Care

Do you put others first and ignore your own needs even to the point of exhaustion? Although enervating, this is quite normal. While many aspects of my life were in turmoil, I felt a profound urgency to take care of everyone else before taking care of me, but I was thoroughly exhausted and frustrated. Feeling overwhelmed, I decided to reach out for help to a friend who is a psychologist. It was the BEST investment I ever made. I sat in front of him, took a breath and realized I had to be honest with someone or I would explode. Full disclosure: I also had to be honest with myself because I wasn't doing that either at that point in time. Slowly I explained what was going on with me physically, and within seconds the words were spilling out of me faster than I could speak. Tears came next, and then the anger and frustration. I completely unloaded on him, finishing with the appeal "And how can I take care of everyone else and ensure they are okay, too?" I wasn't consciously aware of the pressure I had placed on myself to take care of everyone else until that point in time.

He actually gave me permission to think of myself first. He validated my feelings by sharing an article he had written about adversity being a gift in disguise and recognizing the treasure within. During our subsequent sessions I began to comprehend that caring for me was not an act of selfishness and that taking care of others was not my responsibility unless I had the energy to spare and chose to do so. Right then, in my time of need, my one and only job was learning how to care for my body now afflicted with MS. As we focused on new beginnings and the opportunities that were unfolding, he helped me gain the confidence I needed to move forward and the assurance that I would emerge stronger.

When you find yourself with chronic disease, most likely you have not put yourself at the top of your priority list. And as with a car, if you keep driving and never refill the gas tank, eventually you will run out of gas. Remember to refill your tank, fueling your superpowers, and do things that stimulate you and bring you joy.

CHAPTER 18

BE YOUR OWN SUPERHERO

Character cannot be developed in ease and quiet. Only through experiences of trial and suffering can the soul be strengthened, vision cleared, ambition inspired and success achieved.
— Helen Keller

Wow! You've been through quite the rite of passage – thrust unexpectedly into chaos by a trauma, crisis or chronic stress, and undergoing amazing positive transformation as you discovered your superpowers of courage and resilience. But there's one last step: taking an in-depth look inside your heart.

Imagine a staircase going into your heart. As this staircase appears in your mind's eye, take a step down. For reassurance, gently hover your hands above the rails as you descend the smooth white glass steps. Down, down, down you go... suddenly yet gently arriving at the bottom.

At first you are surrounded by darkness, but then light enters the space and a garden is revealed. You can feel the warmth of the sunlight on your face and you feel aglow with its energy.

As you begin to take a few steps deeper into the garden, a feminine divine spirit guide appears. It takes your hand as if to say, "Come with me." Out of the corner of your eye you notice a shadow figure that's masculine, and it distracts you from the spirit guide whose hand you are holding. It sits very still and erect on a bench with its arms stretched wide and resting on the seatback, observing you.

You come upon a body of water that glistens in the sunlight that energizes and comforts you simultaneously. As you kneel down to study your reflection in the water, all you see is sparkling light. When you look a bit upward toward the horizon you simultaneously see the male shadow figure rising from that shimmering light as a form of your masculine divine energy, and become consciously aware that you are the sparkling light. Then the shadow figure appears back on the bench, shifting to one side as if to relax and say, "This is good." It is pleased that you finally see your true self: feminine and masculine divine light together, reflecting brightly in the water.

The time has come to leave your inner heart and ascend the staircase from your heart back to reality. You leave with a new sense of security, knowing that whatever is next in your life journey, all will be okay and you can stop worrying. The shadow on the bench represented the masculine divine presence of God/Spirit/Energy, and your sparkling reflection in the water represented the female divine presence of God/ Spirit/Energy. Your spirit guide helped you bring them together inside you, as you, for complete healing of your body and soul. This is your superhero journey, one that is complete yet incomplete at the same time, proving that you will continue to face challenges that will thrust you into the unknown over and over again. And through that process you will continue to harness the energy within, increasing your confidence while flexing your superpower of resilience.

Few things in life are guaranteed; death and taxes are the only two that come to mind. Yes, someday you will die; and yes, you definitely must pay your taxes in the meantime! In all seriousness, we all have an expiration date; we are just unaware of when it is. So what happens when you find out through a serious diagnosis that your time might be even more limited? Being faced with your mortality is unsettling, to say the least. You lose your sense of self, emotionally and physically, never to be the same person again. Recognizing that you must stop wasting precious time, you put forth the effort to find your passion or purpose based on what you truly value. A diagnosis becomes your wake-up call to living, not merely existing, and turning off the autopilot switch. Instead of suffering in silence, you choose to rejoice in living fully and really being alive.

Some of us don't get life's wake-up call and plod along on autopilot. As we age and grow weary under the weight of chronic stress, small things start to happen to us physically and emotionally. We begin to get hints from the universe that it's time to turn off that autopilot and become present to the world around us.

Life is a journey, not a race to be won or lost. It's a marathon that takes dedication, occasional tweaking and a desire to bring your wellness potential to its pinnacle. There is no crystal ball for predicting what will happen, so you must have a plan for tomorrow while living for today. You must do your best to forgive yourself if you weren't properly prepared, and go with the flow when you come up against something you cannot fight.

Your superhero journey has transformed who you are and how you want to show up in the world. You are no longer completely stressed out while on the endless hamster wheel running in circles trying to grab the proverbial golden carrot that always seems just beyond reach. You have accepted the obstacles in your life as gifts that offer opportunities to learn and grow strong. And you have a deep desire to give back by sharing your new knowledge with others so they can achieve the same sense of self-assurance you have embraced. Your stumbling blocks have become steppingstones leading you through a life well-lived. You have reentered the ordinary world in the context of your new normal, with strength, courage and resilience. You also bring with you your magic elixir: my four-step G.I.F.T. strategic-thinking process that helps you (and others) discover your superpower of resilience.

Recently I was asked, "What if my superhero cape flies off and catches fire?" Yikes! From the previously presented quote by Glenda the Good Witch from *The Wizard of Oz*: "My dear, you always had the power within you." Whether you don a superhero cape or not, you have resiliency within you. You are born with it and all you have to do is be aware of it and develop it; capes are an optional accoutrement.

I am my doctor's favorite conundrum. Although the MRI picture indicates disease activity in my brain, I do not present the associated symptoms. Together we have determined to treat me and not the picture, recognizing that it is more important how I live my life than what my brain looks like in a scan. I listen to and trust my body; my doctor listens to and trusts me. Together we do all we can to keep me well, seeking excellence for my body, and not perfection dictated by others. I ask you to use me, in addition to the several client stories I shared, as living proof that being resilient works, and to give it a try if you haven't already. It might not be a cure per se, but it proves you can live a well life even with chronic disease.

Changing and Learning

Throughout your superhero journey you've adapted to change and gained a greater understanding of and respect for your inner strengths. Throughout your life you will traverse many obstacles, but now you have the confidence to plan for an optimistic future without sacrificing living fully in the present moment. You have acquired a unique set of skills that bring out your superhero powers – those untapped and extraordinary inner strengths that are uniquely yours. And now your mind-body-spirit connection can realize its fullest potential.

What you learned includes shifting how you interpret nutrition, focusing not only on what you eat but why you eat. It is astonishing to realize how normal it is to "eat your emotions," and how much effort it takes to control this so you eat only to satisfy your actual physical hunger.

You have also shifted the way you view exercise, understanding how life-threatening a sedentary lifestyle can be and that exercise includes so much more than simply working out at a gym. Keep in mind this quote from George Bernard Shaw: "We don't stop playing because we grow old; we grow old because we stop playing."

Probably the most important aspect of your superhero journey was learning to release anxiety, decrease stress and discover your deep sense of spirituality that you might have otherwise disregarded. Until you banished stress, you most likely had no idea how overwhelmed your body was by the toxicity of cynicism. It took great effort on your part to pull yourself out of the dark hole of desolation into the divine light of your faith, believe in yourself, believe in a higher power and choose to live fully without sweating the small stuff.

Only through experience can you learn and grow. Sounds super easy, right? Well it's not. You will fall down a lot. But now with the tools of G.I.F.T. you will bravely and powerfully get back up again. Your journey will hopefully be a long one, though you will be tested again and again. Now that you have ignited your superpowers of courage and resilience, you won't give up, nor will you give in. You are strong and you are never alone.

Returning with Your Magic Elixir

As I discussed, resilience is the magic elixir you return with from your superhero journey, and *tikkun olam* is the vehicle by which you help others be extraordinary in their life journeys as well, thereby healing the world. When you successfully cope with challenges in your life it has a ripple effect far beyond you as an individual. By overcoming adversity, recognizing the G.I.F.T. and paying it forward, you become a source of inspiration for others. You show them it's okay to examine their fragile human spirit because when they do they will find their individual superhero qualities. When you share your vulnerability, you afford others permission to be themselves – an often neglected appreciation, and demonstrate and teach the value of empathy over sympathy. When you go from being the student to being the teacher, your journey to learning to live healthfully with chronic disease becomes complete.

Receiving a diagnosis of a chronic illness opened up my soul to the realization of how brief our time here on earth truly is and that we had better make every moment count. My journey has taught me that it is okay to express my belief in the beauty of my soul and the goodness of others. My faith in God/Spirit/Energy and mankind has been renewed over the years and enhances my strength of being, my ability to live my faith and my ability to be my own superhero.

G.I.F.T.

Along with me, you have completed your superhero journey, adjusting to and accepting your new normal. You have learned to cultivate relationships that nurture you rather than drain you. You have found your true purpose or passion so as to become the change you wish to see in the world. You have learned an integrative approach to living a healthy lifestyle that supports your individual needs, and you have raised your energetic vibration. You know what you want to do with your good health. You are able to joyously answer the question "How alive am I willing to be?" You are able to thrive in your new normal that works for you, recognizing that chronic disease does not define you. You can and do live healthfully with it.

Once learned, the four-step G.I.F.T. strategic-thinking process becomes so intrinsic to your thinking that it is automatic, so it's passive, not active. It becomes your WHO –

who you truly are – your core truth – your I AM. YOU as your own superhero! It's your toolkit filled with all of the essential tools for living well. You'll find yourself showing up every day in your life, recognizing the importance of resilience, staying calm in the face of chaos and knowing fully that through struggle and overcoming challenges you become stronger. Be the change you wish to see in the world and set an example for others to follow.

Describe Yourself as a Superhero

To help you visualize what you look like as your own superhero, and to feel more empowered, please complete the statements below. This exercise helps you focus on your strengths – unique only to you – while creating a motto or mantra to recite daily. You might even try taking a physical superpower stance or power pose when you exclaim your daily mantra as an added form of inspiration. Most important, remember to forgive yourself, be gentle with yourself and love yourself. You cannot expect anyone to do that for you until you do it for yourself.

I AM my own superhero.

I AM extraordinary, unleashing my greatness and coming to my own rescue!

My name is: _____

My strengths are: _____

My gremlin is: _____

My superhero powers that battle my gremlin are: _____

_____

My superhero motto is: _____

One word that is my affirmation or superpower word is:

_____

Using this word in each of the following statements, I affirm that:

I think _____ thoughts.

I speak _____ words.

I take _____ actions.

I AM _____!

Remember, it takes 30 days to change a habit and 90 days to make it stick. So be sure to give yourself plenty of time to reap the full benefits of all that you've learned.

Your superhero journey takes a circular path. By facing constant challenges, changing, learning and growing as you embark on each steppingstone to success, you become keenly aware of your courage, strength and resilience. Pause for a moment to congratulate yourself on how far you've come and what you've achieved, for this has not been an easy task. Know you will be tested again. That is a natural part of life. Yet as you reflect on where you've been and what you've overcome, moving forward and facing new challenges will no longer seem as insurmountable. In the face of chaos you will knowingly whisper to yourself, "Panic," remembering the Panic Game and G.I.F.T. You'll confidently know you've got this as you call on your superpower of resilience.

To all those afflicted with chronic disease or dis-ease: you are not alone.

Be present.

Be purposeful.

Be well.

Be Your Own Superhero!

No hero's journey ever ends, and your next adventure is already happening. The moment you accept the call to adventure, the road of trials begins finding its way from your unconscious awareness into your consciousness, freeing and expanding your imagination, helping you become the healing you hope to create.
– Martha Beck

SUGGESTED RESOURCES

Books:

Live in Wellness Now: A Proactive Guide to Living Well (March 2013) by Barbara B. Appelbaum

The Complete Vision Board Kit: Using the Power of Intention and Visualization to Achieve Your Dreams (October 2008) by John Assaraf

Finding Your Way in a Wild New World: Reclaim Your True Nature to Create the Life You Want (January 2013) by Martha Beck

Canyon Ranch 30 Days to a Better Brain: A Groundbreaking Program for Improving Your Memory, Concentration, Mood, and Overall Well-Being (May 2014) by Richard Carmona

Taming Your Gremlin: A Surprisingly Simple Method for Getting Out of Your Own Way (July 2003) by Rick Carson

Meditations from the Mat: Daily Reflections on the Path of Yoga (December 2002) by Rolf Gates and Katrina Kenison

Healing with God's Love: Kabbalah's Hidden Secrets (January 2015) by Douglas Goldhamer and Peggy Bagley

10% Happier: How I Tamed the Voice in My Head, Reduced Stress without Losing My Edge, and Found Self-Help That Actually Works (December 2014) by Dan Harris

We Plan, God Laughs: What to Do When Life Hits You Over the Head (June 2009) by Sherre Hirsch

When Breath Becomes Air (January 2016) by Paul Kalanithi and Abraham Verghese

When Bad Things Happen to Good People (August 2004) by Harold S. Kushner

Science of Breath: A Practical Guide (January 2007) by Swami Rama, Dr. Rudolph Ballentine and Dr. Alan Hymes

Your Body Speaks Your Mind: Decoding the Emotional, Psychological, and Spiritual Messages That Underlie Illness (April 2006) by Deb Shapiro

2 Weeks to a Younger Brain: An Innovative Program for a Better Memory and Sharper Mind (April 2016) by Gary Small and Gigi Vorgan

Aging with Grace: What the Nun Study Teaches Us about Leading Longer, Healthier, and More Meaningful Lives (May 2002) by David Snowdon

The Energy Healing Experiments: Science Reveals Our Natural Power to Heal (August 2008) by Gary E. Schwartz

Websites:

AARP – http://www.aarp.org

Alzheimer's Association – http://www.alz.org

Andrew Weil, MD – https://www.drweil.com

The Global Consciousness Project – http://noosphere.princeton.edu

Centers for Disease Control and Prevention, Healthy Aging – https://www.cdc.gov/aging/index.html

Institute for Integrative Nutrition – www.integrativenutrition.com

The Laboratory for Advances in Consciousness and Health at the University of Arizona – http://lach.web.arizona.edu

Mindful magazine – http://www.mindful.org/magazine

Modern Day MS – http://moderndayms.com

National MS Society – www.nationalmssociety.org

University of Arizona Center for Integrative Medicine – https://integrativemedicine.arizona.edu

Smartphone Apps:

Apple or Samsung Health

Calm

JEFIT

Lumosity

Mango Health

Medsafe

My Fitness Pal

Pandora "Healing Earth" Radio

Pocket Yoga

Relax Melodies: Sleep Sounds, White Noise & Fan by iLBSoft

Sleep Pillow Sounds

WebMD

NOTES

1. Sari Harrar, "Health: What to Expect in Your 50s: Plus, Ways to Pamper Your Heart," *AARP The Magazine*, June/July 2017, https://www.aarp.org/health/healthy-living/info-2017/over-50-healthy-living-tips.html

2. "About Chronic Conditions," National Health Council, 3/21/16, http://www.nationalhealthcouncil.org/newsroom/about-chronic-conditions

3. World Health Organization's constitutional principles, http://www.who.int/about/mission/en

4. "About Wellness," National Wellness Institute, http://www.nationalwellness.org/?page=AboutWellness

5. "Chronic Disease," MedicineNet.com, https://www.medicinenet.com/script/main/art.asp?articlekey=33490

6. "Chronic Disease Overview," Centers for Disease Control and Prevention, https://www.cdc.gov/chronicdisease/overview/index.htm

7. "About Chronic Diseases," National Health Council, 7/29/14, http://www.nationalhealthcouncil.org/sites/default/files/NHC_Files/Pdf_Files/AboutChronicDisease.pdf

8. "Understanding the Stress Response: Chronic Activation of this Survival Mechanism Impairs Health," Harvard Health

Publishing/Harvard Medical School, updated 3/18/16; published March 2011, https://www.health.harvard.edu/staying-healthy/understanding-the-stress-response

9. Martha Chalnick, "Reserves of Resilience," January 7, 2016, https://marlachalnick.com/category/uncategorized/page/2

10. Andrew Weil, "Video: Breathing Exercises: 4-7-8 Breath," https://www.drweil.com/videos-features/videos/breathing-exercises-4-7-8-breath

11. Drenna Waldrop-Valverde, "Cognitive and Affective Issues in Chronic Disease: Effects on Self-Management," National Institutes of Health Office of Behavioral and Social Sciences Research, 9/9/15, https://obssr.od.nih.gov/cognitive-and-affective-issues-in-chronic-disease-effects-on-self-management/

12. John E. Morley, "Cognition and Chronic Disease," *Journal of Post-Acute and Long-term Care Medicine*, May 1, 2017, vol. 18, issue 5, http://www.jamda.com/article/S1525-8610(17)30105-6/fulltext

13. "The Mind-Body Connection . . . Between Stress and Disease," Personal Safety Nets.org, http://www.personalsafetynets.org/mind-body-connection-between-stress-and-disease

14. National MS Society News Update, January 13, 2017, https://www.nationalmssociety.org/About-the-Society/News/New-Study-Resilience-in-People-with-Chronic-Disea

15. "What Is Alzheimer's?," Alzheimer's Association, https://www.alz.org/alzheimers_disease_what_is_alzheimers.asp

16. Gary Small and Gigi Vorgan, *2 Weeks to a Younger Brain*, 2016, Boca Raton, FL: Humanix Books

17. Mark Wheeler, "Evidence Builds that Meditation Strengthens the Brain, UCLA Researchers Say," UCLA Newsroom, March 14, 2012, http://newsroom.ucla.edu/releases/evidence-builds-that-meditation-230237

18. Alice Calaprice, *Dear Professor Einstein: Albert Einstein's Letters to and from Children*, 2002, Amherst, NY: Prometheus Books

19. "ACSM Certified Clinical Exercise Physiologist®," https://certification.acsm.org/acsm-certified-clinical-exercise-physiologist

20. "Survey Reveals Current Trends in Men's Health," NewsUSA, 5/31/07, http://www.newsusa.com/articles/article/survey-reveals-current-trends-in-mens-health.aspx

21. "Overweight & Obesity Statistics," National Institutes of Health – National Institute of Diabetes and Kidney Diseases, August 2017, https://www.niddk.nih.gov/health-information/health-statistics/overweight-obesity

22. Marie T. Brown and Jennifer K. Bussell, "Medication Adherence: WHO Cares?," *Mayo Clinic Proceedings*, April 2011, 86(4): 304–314, doi: 10.4065/mcp.2010.0575, PMCID: PMC3068890, https://www.ncbi.nlm.nih.gov/pmc/articles/PMC3068890

ACKNOWLEDGMENTS

Thanks to:

- My Uncle Emil for telling stories of being a mycologist with Dr. Andrew Weil, and for turning me on to Dr. Weil's integrative approach to wellness when I was a young girl

- Lynne Klippel for her love, guidance, and professional support

- My friends and clients, who will remain anonymous, who allowed me to use their stories in support of the tools I am teaching

- My family and friends, who always support my endeavors to make a positive difference in the world

- And, most important, my parents, for exemplifying what it truly means to be your own superhero

ABOUT THE AUTHOR

Barbara B. Appelbaum, PCC, MBA, MAT

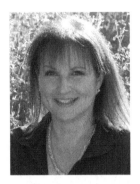

As a motivational speaker, published author, certified wellness coach and consultant, Barbara inspires people to look and feel younger longer, even with a chronic illness, through mindful health and a meaningful life. She is recognized as an expert in the growing field of an integrative approach to proactive wellness. Her first book was *Live in Wellness Now,* published by Love your Life Publishing in 2013.

Barbara is a seasoned professional who authentically walks her talk every day. In a matter of mere seconds on a Thursday morning in June of 2006, her life changed forever. In the blink of an eye she experienced symptoms of what appeared to be a stroke at the mere age of 44. She ultimately received a diagnosis of multiple sclerosis. This trauma became the gift that transformed everything, making her realize the importance of living life healthfully and intentionally while helping others do the same, especially as they age.

Barbara's genuine compassion, expertise and firsthand knowledge educate and inspire motivated middle-aged professionals to stave off age-related disease and learn to be present, be purposeful and be well. By combining an integrative approach to nutrition, spirituality and neuroscience principles, she helps people understand how to be proactive in their health care versus reactionary in their sick care so they can feel great in their bodies and in their lives. Her greatest wish is to never hear a person say, "I should be taking better care of myself."

As a member of the National Speaker's Association, Barbara holds two master's degrees, one in business and one in teaching, and is a certified member of the International Coach Federation, International Association for Health Coaches, and American Association of Drugless Practitioners. She is a Certified Wellness Coach and Certified Integrative Nutrition Health Coach. She is also a consultant to the National Multiple Sclerosis Society and an Ambassador for the National MS Society – Greater Illinois Chapter. She guest-lectures regularly at Canyon Ranch in Tucson, Arizona, and is a contributor to the Modern Day MS blog.

Ways to contact Barbara include:

Website: www.appelbaumwellness.com

Facebook: www.facebook.com/appelbaumwellnessllc

LinkedIn: www.linkedin.com/in/barbarabappelbaum

Made in the USA
San Bernardino, CA
16 May 2018